Searching for a Zebra

SEARCHING for a Zebra

MONICA HARE

This is a true story.
It shouldn't be, but it is. But that's not
the shocking part, which is that many
people have stories like ours.
And that is why I wrote it.
I don't want to be sued so some names have been
changed, and I recreated dialogue, but **the story is true**.

Also,
I am not a doctor.
Everyone's experience is different.
Researchers are learning more every day.
This is our family's story.
The opinions are my own.

ISBN: 979-8-218-36830-2
Library of Congress Control Number: 2024903302

DEDICATION

To every person who has a rare disorder

&

To the people who love them

Table of Contents

THANK YOU

- ♡ To Dr. "Avery" for realizing Myles had a fever disorder, and for not giving up
- ♡ To the doctor who diagnosed Myles and is still working to help him
- ♡ To Caleb for saying, *You should write a book.*
- ♡ To Shawn for being my best friend and for loving our children so, so much.
- ♡ To my kids for being supportive and doing all they could to help when Myles got sick
- ♡ To my mom and sister and brother-in-law for always answering when we needed them
- ♡ Most importantly, thank you, God.

CHAPTER ONE

There's a chance you're going to think I'm crazy when you start reading this.

Does the name "Gypsy Rose" ring a bell? In case you aren't familiar, Gypsy talked her boyfriend into brutally murdering her mother in 2015. She had endured years of medical torture—unneeded medication, a feeding tube, having her head shaved (the last one was not necessarily medical, but would definitely be considered torture for a young teenage girl)—all a result of her mama's Munchausen by proxy. (Fun fact: it isn't called Munchausen by proxy anymore. Now it's *Factitious Disorder Imposed on Another*. I have no idea why they changed it, but I do think the new name is kind of catchy.)

By my son's first birthday, I had taken him to a doctor's office (or to a hospital emergency room) twenty-three times. To put that into perspective, there are 12 months in a year. I took him to see a physician, on average, twice a month. During that first year, he had a multitude of throat swabs and flu tests. All of those were negative. And please don't think for one second I slowed down that second year of his life. That was the year of the Coronavirus, so of course we added to the tally. From the time he turned one until his second birthday, we made close to fifty trips to see doctors.

So, are you thinking *she must be a nervous first-time mom*? I wasn't (the first-time mom part, anyway). Myles is my *fifth* child. Am I a crazy person? Well, that depends on who you ask. But not crazy like Gypsy's mom. I humbly ask that you keep an open mind as you trek down this path with me. My hope and prayer is that Myles' story, *our* story, will help someone else to have an easier journey. Perhaps reach a quicker diagnosis. Ideally, acquire treatment sooner. But even if you have a different outcome (or you're on a different journey altogether), maybe this will give you hope in whatever you're going through. And if you don't have any problems or struggles, medical or otherwise, maybe you'll just enjoy reading about our experience in navigating the best and the worst of the dreaded--but necessary--

medical system. (Also, please send me an email and tell me how you do it--get through life with no problems, I mean.)

The stark white walls of the exam room close me in as I realize this is our third time sitting in this room—or one just like it—this month. I am holding my very hot sleeping baby—last I checked, his temp was just over 104. Being in a doctor's office, strangely enough, usually allowed me to relax just a little. If he had a febrile seizure at least they'd know what to do. I wouldn't be alone. But when I think of the number of times we've been here lately, I tense up again. Myles is resting, but I know it won't last. Pretty soon—when we hear the knock on the wooden door—the silence will be replaced with his cries. We've been through this so many times. He doesn't realize they're trying to help him, and he just wants to be left alone, safe in my arms. As soon as they start poking and prodding him, he will wake up and go into defense mode.

The heat radiating from his little body makes us sticky with sweat.

Knock. Knock. Knock.

Three quick raps on the door. His tiny body jerks awake.

Helloooo. Got a sick little fella today?

Here we go again...

REWIND

I should probably give you a little bit of history. I was 38 years old and I had an 18-year-old daughter, Hailey, and three sons: Caleb, who was 17 (Irish twins—when Hailey was four months old, I learned I was almost three months pregnant with Caleb), Cash was 7, and my baby...Max. Maxie was only 3 and he was a firecracker right from the start! But the baby is supposed to be, right? I was an older mother, compared to when I had Hailey and Caleb anyway, and by the time you've had that many babies you realize how fast the time goes and you cherish every moment. So Max was my baby—*our* baby—and we treated him as such. He got away with a little more. And he had (and still has) a dynamic personality. Max makes us laugh. He is full of energy, and so creative!

I was always pretty judgmental when I saw parents letting their children misbehave in public. Max was the one who taught me to be less critical and more compassionate toward those same parents. He was never *bad*—just more energetic, curious, lively...fun.

So, we had our big kids who were almost grown, Cash, who was born ready to be a big brother, and our sweet Maxie—the "baby."

Back then, I was happy to be teaching second grade as a long-term substitute at our local pre- through second grade primary school. I had taught school when Hailey and Caleb were younger, and I subbed a little at their high school when they were older, but I was finally, officially, getting back into teaching. There was even a rumor that a full-time teaching position might become available before my long-term placement was up. I felt settled and content for the first time in a while.

Now this is a little (well, a lot) off-topic, but when I was a little girl, I had an older cousin who had a boyfriend. They had dated for several years and were in *love*. Even at my age I could see that he was pretty hot. My cousin had also dated his (even hotter) older brother before she dated him—just a couple of dates, nothing serious, but still it was like a romance novel or a soap opera to twelve-year-old me. Well, cute boyfriend eventually broke up with her and it was devastating...first-love heartbreak. Months later, after she started eating again, my cousin met her future husband, but early into her and future-husband's courtship a very handsome Navy man started asking her out and trying to woo her with dozens of roses and expensive gifts. He even proposed (which she promptly turned down) with a big diamond ring and two dozen roses. I thought she was living a storybook life! I remember thinking, *Wow! I hope my life is like that.* Passion! Excitement!

What I didn't know at the time was that my life would be *very* exciting. I also didn't realize that *excitement* is not the same as *happiness*. My life has been an adventure, and I can't tell you how many times my mind wanders back to my aspirations as a twelve-year-old to have a storybook existence. There have been times, through the years, I have experienced pain that I would not wish on another soul. But I have also been blessed more than I could have ever imagined: my children, my husband, becoming a Christian... And I would go through all the bad again if I had to, just to have the good.

My point, from that little detour we just took together, is that at that time in my life, I was content. But God must have thought I needed a little more excitement.

A LITTLE MORE EXCITEMENT

I peed on a stick. (Don't the best things in life start out like that?) Cash and Max were playing in the living room, and I didn't want to sit and watch the pink shadow drift across the testing window, so I went to play with them while the timer ran down. I hadn't had a period in months, and I was on a low-dose birth control pill (low-dose because I was still breastfeeding Maxie), so it was *highly* unlikely that I was pregnant. I only took the test because I had been having some nausea like I had when I was newly pregnant with my other four and I wanted to make sure, as unlikely as it was.

But when I went back into the restroom and saw those two lines, I knew. All of the impossibilities faded away instantly. (By the way, if anyone ever tells you that you can't get pregnant while you're breastfeeding, laugh at them. I've done it three times.) With all of my previous pregnancies, I took multiple tests. I doubted each one. But, somehow, I just knew that this test was right...I was going to have another precious little baby. Maybe it took those first four times for me to believe that a positive pregnancy test means you're probably going to have a baby? But it was actually more than that...I just *knew.* I was pregnant. At 39. With baby number five.

God was blessing us with a sweet, innocent little life. After all the joy he had given us with Hailey, Caleb, Cash, and little Maxie, he was sending us another precious little baby to love.

I cried.

And by *cried*, I mean I broke down on the bathroom floor—quietly. I didn't want the boys to hear me. I was curled up into the fetal position, my body racked with sobs, but I didn't make a sound (unless you count when I would gasp for air). You know when your heart feels like it's been ripped out, but you still have to portray a calm, sane person to everyone around you? That's what I was trying to do. I didn't want the boys—or anyone else—to know. I was so scared. I was afraid of what my family would say. I was afraid of what my husband would say. I was afraid I wouldn't get that rumored teaching position... Who would want to hire someone who would have to take off for maternity leave (not to mention, the *many* doctor appointments leading up to that) their first year? But mostly? I cried because I felt like I would never be able to give enough love and affection to this new little baby, while still giving my other children the care they deserved, and the attention and time I wanted to give all of them. Am I ashamed now, looking back, that I didn't have enough faith to be thrilled about the new little life inside me? Yes. Of course, I am. But that's what happened, and it is one of many examples where God did something amazing, when I thought all was lost.

I couldn't tell anyone. I literally *could not say the words*. Shawn was at work when I took the test, and he knew something was wrong when he got home. Not only were my eyes swollen, but he could just tell something was off. He asked me what was going on, and I wanted to tell him, but I couldn't say it.

This man knew everything about me. He knew my worst fears, my thoughts on everything from politics to the best way to fold towels (half, half again, then thirds—unless you're putting them in a basket, then you roll them). Shawn had heard me rant about anything and everything that had ever bothered me and knew how to make me smile when I was mad at the world. But I just couldn't tell him. His concern about my strange mood made the worries start cycling through my head again, so back I went to cry on the bathroom floor, for the second time that day. Surprisingly, that second round of sobbing (silently) in the bathroom gave me an idea.

I didn't have to tell him. I could just let him find out on his own! I got the box out of the trash can. I put the test on the bathroom counter. We kept our countertop pretty free of clutter back then, so the positive pregnancy test would be impossible to miss. Shawn would see it. He would know I was pregnant with baby number 5. It didn't change any of the facts of the situation, but I wouldn't have to tell him myself, and he could have some time to process it before we talked.

My brilliant plan would work. Except that I forgot one thing: my husband is a human man. I'm not saying men aren't smart, or observant, or thoughtful. My husband is all of those things. But, sometimes, I need him to be a little more than an ordinary human man. I need him to be a mind-reader. On those occasions, I expect him to look around, take in all the clues, consider my current mood, and make the appropriate deduction. In this case, leaving a positive pregnancy test in an obvious place was not enough for him to come to the correct conclusion.

Two days later, Shawn still hadn't mentioned the test on the counter. My nerves were shot. I felt like I was a guilty criminal, and my home was the interrogation room.

(But no one was asking the right questions.) There was no escape—and I *craved* the sweet relief of confession—but saying it out loud would make it real. Ever watch a police interrogation and the cops are like, *Come on, you'll feel so much better when you confess!*

Okay... Okay, I confess.

Now, do you feel that? That huge weight being lifted off your shoulders?

Yeah. Yeah, I do. I can finally breathe again. I feel so free!

Good. Now turn around and put your hands behind your back.

As long as no one else knew that the test was positive, it could just be my imagination. I didn't have to deal with the consequences. I waivered between wanting everyone to know and wanting no one to know.

The straw that broke the camel's back came when my sweet, caring husband had been trying to figure out why I was acting *weird* for over 48 hours, and he made a comment of something to the effect of, W*hat's wrong with you?* Considering I was a tiny bit high-strung from keeping this life-changing secret, paired with the fact that I was sure that he had seen (and comprehended the meaning of) the positive pregnancy test and was upset about it, I broke down in tears. I didn't even make it to the bathroom floor this time.

Apparently, I had given my husband too much credit when I assumed he would see the *positive pregnancy test* on our bathroom counter and say, H*ey! I think someone in this house is pregnant and since my wife is the only female who lives here, it must be her.*

He did not have a clue. Bless his heart.

Through tears, I blurted out, Y*ou know what's wrong with me!*

He didn't.

So, I told him. The words finally spilled out. I told him that in a few months, he was going to have another child.

My entire body braced for his reaction. My eyes, clouded with tears, were focused on a spot on the floor—I wanted to look anywhere but at the disappointment on his face.

I was still looking down when I heard him go, *huh*. You know that sound you make when you've figured something out? Like, *Huh. I never knew that before*. That's the sound he made. So I looked up. He was smiling. Then as I finally looked in his eyes, my 48-year-old husband giggled--like a schoolgirl.

That's why you've been so upset lately?

To say he was ecstatic would be putting it mildly. He pulled me into his arms and told me everything was going to be okay. He said, *Look at our kids. This one is going to be amazing, just like the others.* Shawn loves his children. He already knew he was going to love this baby as much as the others. And he convinced me that I had enough love (and energy) for this new baby and our other children, too. And while I can tell you that we absolutely did, we had no idea what was coming.

SNIPS AND SNAILS AND PUPPY DOG TAILS

Jump ahead a few months, and I'm a little larger and a lot more exhausted. Being pregnant at 39 was different than being pregnant at 20. Or 21. Or even 31 or 35. You get the idea. I was teaching kindergarten (turns out the rumor about the full-time position was true—and they hired me!), being a mom, and growing a little boy. Did I mention I was very tired?

Now, I know there are some strong, confident women who were pregnant at 40 who are going to say, *I had a great pregnancy! I danced through those nine months like it was my quinceañera!* Great! Good for you! I am truly, sincerely happy that you had that beautiful journey to motherhood. That was not my experience.

I have always had Braxton Hicks contractions with my pregnancies, but they were really intense with this one. If I was standing (and I'm *always* standing when I'm teaching) my stomach was rock hard. And not in an abs of steel kind of way. Eventually, my doctor told me I needed to stay home and stay off my feet. We wanted to keep Itty

Bear (our nickname for him) on the inside for as long as possible.

Besides the early contractions (and pretty severe morning sickness—or more accurately, *all-day sickness that lasted six months*) my pregnancy went well.

I had been closely monitored due to being labeled a "geriatric pregnancy"—being an *older* mother. (Just what I wanted to see on my medical chart at every single checkup.) Fortunately, despite my elderly condition, my baby boy seemed to be healthy and growing as expected.

I went in for an induction at 39 weeks. I had a very sweet nurse midwife who, despite my begging around week 37, would not induce me for another two weeks. Shawn and I made the 45-minute drive to the hospital (the same one where Cash and Max were born) as the sun was rising. I had invited Hailey to be at the birth this time, and I told her to take her time making the drive there. Even though I've always had speedy labor and deliveries, it takes a while to get things going, then at least a couple of hours of contractions. But as soon as they started the Pitocin, I asked Shawn to call Hailey and tell her she would need to come on to the hospital if she wanted to make it to the birth. It was not going to be long. Fortunately, she was already almost there, because *he* was almost there, too. Apparently, all of those early contractions had helped get me ready. At 9:37 a.m., Myles River Dean Hare made his grand entrance like he does everything: rapidly and dramatically.

Myles River. The one we had no idea we needed and can't imagine life before he was part of our's. He had all of our hearts right from the beginning. He was like sunshine and a fresh summer rain mixed together. But even that doesn't describe him. How do you describe a newborn baby? It's the most wonderful thing in this world, so there's nothing to really compare it to. You know the smell? The fresh, sweet smell of a newborn? I would hold him close to my skin, breathing him in. Smoothing his soft hair with my fingers while he nursed. Babies are a precious gift from God. Myles was like that extra gift hiding behind the couch on Christmas morning. I had thought my baby days were over. I held onto this one tightly.

I met my husband when I was working in the daycare his sister helped operate. I was sitting in the nursery holding one of the babies the first time he spoke to me. Shawn had walked by, and he looked at me and said, *That's the best job in the world right there*. Now I was holding one of *his* babies, and it absolutely was the best job in the world.

When Myles was three weeks old, I reluctantly returned to work. Teachers don't get maternity leave in

Kentucky (that's a whole 'nother story), and I had used up all of my sick days (I didn't have many as a first-year teacher, anyway) so I couldn't really afford to stay home any longer. I pumped during my planning and I snuck home on my lunch break to nurse him. I had always stayed home with my babies until they were older, so leaving him for hours at a time at his age was heart-wrenching. I kept telling myself, *you just have to make it until summer*. Of course, *summer* lasts only a couple of months then I would have to leave him again, but positive thinking got me through the next few weeks.

Myles completed our family. Most of my babies have been surprises. When you are blessed like that, it can be scary at first, but as soon as you lay eyes on that precious little baby, it's like your heart literally grows. I can't explain it, but it's the most wonderful feeling in the world.

I thank God every day for our kids. They each have such unique personalities and bring so much joy to our lives. Myles added a whole new layer. My favorite thing to do is to watch my children interact with each other. Max, who had just gone from *the baby* to *the middle child*, transitioned into the best big brother. He would hug Myles and say, *you're the cutest baby ever*. Cash was my helper. Anything Myles or I needed, he was on top of it. He wanted to hold Myles anytime his dad or I didn't have him. He even won the heart of his big brother, Caleb. Caleb's always been more interested in playing with his brothers when they're big enough to throw a ball around, but Myles' quick smile and vibrant personality was quick to captivate him. Hailey stayed busy with school and work at the University of Kentucky, but she came to see her new baby brother when she could. She had stayed the night with us at the hospital, and it broke her heart when she had to leave him to go back to Lexington. Her favorite new hobby was buying tiny, little clothes.

Myles was healthy, happy, and very alert from day one. He also had a sparkle of mischievousness in his eyes. We had seen some of that in Max, but Myles' was a little...more. When Max was four months old, he tried to pull up to an end table, fell, and got a cut over his eye that left a scar. When he was two, he decided to hide in a dryer (closing himself inside) and giving me a near-panic attack as I searched for him. Thankfully I noticed that the dryer door was closed, and it had been open as I had just carried a load of clothes to the living room to fold. He was only in there for about two minutes, and when I opened the door he wasn't scared or crying. He had a big smile on his face. Max has always been quick with a laugh, outgoing, and needs just a teeny tiny bit of *direction* at times. Well, Myles had that same sparkle in his eyes like his big brother, Max. But like I said, it was *more*.

Suffice it to say, Myles River has always kept us on our toes. I can't tell you how many times someone has said to us, *if only we could bottle that energy*...which I know is a polite way of saying *don't you know how to control your child?* Remember how I said Max was the one who taught me to be more compassionate toward other parents? He did. He made me more understanding that sometimes parents are doing everything they can to teach their child how to act. Some kids just have a little more spunk...a lot more energy...and their parents are actually trying their best. But even though I had learned to be more compassionate, I was still aware that others were judging *me*. I still felt the need to tell strangers, *he's the baby*, as if that absolved me of my inability to force compliance in my son. But then Max *wasn't* the baby anymore. And that streak of "energy" was nothing compared to the spontaneous roller-coaster tornado that is Myles.

If you drove by my house, it would be a normal sight to see Myles on top of something—like my Explorer (so far, he hasn't figured out how to get on the roof of the house...but it's coming). Then again, you might see him chasing one of his brothers with a water gun. You might overhear him proposing marriage to one of the (older) neighbor girls. Or to his big brother's girlfriend (whom he admits to having a *big crush* on). Itty has a big personality and (when he feels good) energy that doesn't stop. He's been like that since day one.

From the time he was born, Myles has brought indescribable joy into our lives. He was the piece that only God knew we needed. We felt like we had already been so blessed, then God blessed us some more with this fun, boisterous little bundle of happiness. He would go, go, go full throttle. So when he got sick, it was like the earth had been pushed off its' axis. It was not normal. Myles went from *go, go, go* to lying listlessly in my arms for days.

A VIRUS?

He was three months and two days old. We had been taking him to a pediatric nurse practitioner who had recently started practicing in our town for his well-child checkups. A good friend of mine from church worked with her at the time, so I had full confidence that he was in good hands with both of them. And besides, Myles was healthy, energetic, and nursing like a champ.

When his fever started rising, I called the doctor's office to get him in as soon as possible. He was so little, and so hot.

We took him in, and she checked him out from head to toe. Looked in his mouth...checked his ears...listened to his heart and lungs. His lymph nodes were swollen, but everything else seemed okay. The nurse did strep and flu tests. Both were negative.

It looks like he's got his first virus. Give him 2.5 milliliters of infants Tylenol every four hours.

With instructions to come back in if his condition worsened or we couldn't get his temp down, we were on our way.

If I was a first-time mom, I probably would've been a lot more freaked out than I was. But as Myles was my fifth baby, I understood that little ones get sick sometimes. And a fever is the body's way of stimulating your immune system so it makes it harder for viruses and bacteria to thrive and survive. So although I *really* didn't like that my baby was sick and feeling miserable, I understood that this was just temporary, and he would be happy and healthy in a couple of days. And he was.

After about two days, Myles made a full recovery. He was back to 110% (I know 100 is actually, technically, the highest percentage he could be, but it sure seemed like 110% compared to where he was in the days before). He was laughing and playing, and his temperature was completely normal.

This blissful moment in time spanned exactly two weeks and two days.

When Myles was three months, three weeks, and six days old he started running a fever, again. Why was this baby sick? He didn't go to daycare. He didn't participate in any risky activities—no smoking or wild parties for my boy. I was home with the kids for the summer, so he was mostly around me, his dad, and his brothers. We went to church two or three times a week but didn't pass him around—if I wasn't holding him his Aunt MeMe was. Oh, and the breastmilk he was drinking was full of antibodies. What more could I do to keep my baby healthy?

His temperature quickly rose to 104°. He was tiny and hot and his dad had a history of febrile seizures. It was a Saturday, so we bypassed our small local hospital and quickly drove the 33 miles to the hospital he was born in. They, at least, had a pediatric wing. We felt like that was our best option.

They checked him out. They listened to his heart and lungs. They did all the things they do when a baby is running a fever. They asked, "What are his symptoms?" *He's lethargic. He has a very high temperature.* It could literally be anything. The doctor said his ears kind of looked a little off. When everything came back negative, he was diagnosed with otitis media—an ear infection—and prescribed his first round of antibiotics.

This time, he didn't get over it in two days. On Monday, he was still running a fever. Now (because of the antibiotics) he also had diarrhea. What he was not doing was pulling at his ears. Or screaming in pain. All my other children had ear infections at least once (three of the four had so many they got tubes), and the common denominator of those experiences was the screaming. They hurt. They would cry that ear-shrieking sound that let you know they were in pain. Myles wasn't doing that. He was just limp. He was weak and hot and I wanted to do anything I could to make him feel better.

We made another appointment with his nurse practitioner.

I carried him in wearing just a diaper. The heat radiating off his little body scared me. At home we had been putting cool washcloths under his arms and on the back of his neck. It didn't help a whole lot, but we had to do *something*.

His nurse seemed a little taken aback when she placed the pulse oximeter on his tiny finger and first touched his skin. Her concern made my stomach drop.

Myles' nurse practitioner knocked gently on the door before walking into the room. I explained how his temp had suddenly shot up early Saturday morning, and all about our visit to the ER. She carefully examined him in my arms as he slept. He twitched when she placed the cold metal disk of the stethoscope on his chest, but that was the only reaction he had to being handled.

After retesting him for flu and strep and doing all the necessary poking and prodding, we didn't really get any definitive answers. She said the diarrhea was most likely from taking amoxicillin and suggested we give him probiotics to offset that. She thought he probably had another virus. I was surprised she didn't mention his ears.

How did his ears look today? The doctor at the hospital said he needed the antibiotics for his ear infection, but he hasn't acted like his ears bother him at all.

I was curious about how they were today. Did he *really* need the amoxicillin?

His ears looked fine...but let me take another look.

She took her time looking into both ears before announcing they looked great.

I've never really been skeptical of doctors, but Myles' symptoms combined with his nurse practitioner's proclamation that his ears were fine did make me question his previous diagnosis. It was possible that his ears had healed since he was seen at the emergency room, but if the infection was bad enough for antibiotics wouldn't they still be a little pink at least? I looked at his visit notes and his NP had written *normal form and location|TM's pearly gray*. I needed to know what *TM's* were and *were they supposed to be pearly gray? Was that good or bad?* A quick search online told me that *TM* is short for *tympanic membrane*, which is the technical term for *eardrum*. When I searched *tympanic membrane color* it literally said *pearly gray* in large font at the top of the results. So why did the doctor at the emergency room diagnose him with an ear infection?

KILL, KILL, KILL

the germs

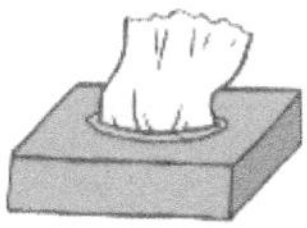

So now I'm confused, worried, and very concerned about my Itty. It sounds like we are probably dealing with another virus. How is this baby getting sick? While I am most certainly not a doctor, it doesn't take years of medical school training to know that viruses are passed from person to person. You need to come in contact with germs in order to catch a virus. As I said earlier, we had been keeping Myles at home. I was treasuring every second of summer vacation, and about 95 percent of the time I had Myles snuggled in my arms.

We were doing everything we could think of to keep Itty healthy. But we weren't literally keeping him in a bubble. His big sister and oldest brother went to college and their part-time jobs, so when they visited there was a possibility of spreading germs. His (younger) big brothers played with the neighbor girls and with church friends, lending another avenue for germs to travel. His daddy and aunts and uncles all went to work. So it was not impossible for Myles to have a virus. Eventually, I accepted that there were actually several ways he had been exposed, so his dad and I just made a commitment to do better.

We would clean more. Use more bleach. Limit his exposure to others—even more than we already had. We would protect Myles River from *all* the germs.

And our plan would have worked...*if it weren't for those meddling kids.*

Well...that's kind of a stretch, but I've always wanted to say it. And it was *sort of* because of kids. I mean, it wasn't intentional, but...

Let me explain.

School was now officially back in session.

I don't know how familiar you are with kindergarten, so I'll tell you a little about the beginning of the year. Some of these kids have never been away from their parents. They have never attended daycare or preschool. Maybe mom or dad stayed home with them, or maybe they had an aunt to look after them while their parents worked. This affected our situation in two ways:

1. Children who have not been around many other children do not have a great immunity response and tend to get sick—often—during the first weeks of kindergarten. As Shawn and I have just declared war on germs, this is like being thrown into the middle of

Ukraine and Russia. But with germs. Instead of weapons. Does that make sense?

2. These little guys who have not been away from mommy and daddy are going to have a bit of an adjustment period. There are tears, and with those tears come runny noses. What do runny noses carry? Germs.

These precious little germ monsters need lots of extra love and affection to get them through this new phase in their lives where they are learning to cope with separation from their parents. Sometimes, I am used as a Kleenex. And that's okay—I believe teaching these little guys that there are people in the world (besides mom and dad) who love them and care about meeting their needs is one of the most important and meaningful parts of my job. But it also means that I am now a germ transportation factory.

There is one other thing that I haven't mentioned yet about the beginning of kindergarten: it is exhausting. When I say it is exhausting, I want to be clear. I don't mean that when you get home from school you will be tired. I don't mean that you may want to take a nap before you cook supper and check your kids' backpacks, have them do homework, and choose their outfits for tomorrow. I mean that you are so tired that you want to crawl into a quiet space where there is no sound and zero visual stimulation, and then stay in that magical place for 48 hours. But you can't. Because you have to do all of the other things I mentioned before: the cooking, the homework, and the preparation for tomorrow. Only after all of that can you try to get in bed a little early, then wake up a few times to nightmares about forgetting to submit attendance on time or kids accidentally missing their bus. Then, before you know it, it's almost time for your first alarm to go off so you just get out of bed and start the day. This goes on for two weeks.

After two weeks the kids magically figure out that school is a fun and happy place to be. After two weeks, my students have practiced and learned our rules and expectations. After two weeks, the whole kindergarten class settles into a routine, and you (the teacher) go from mind-numbing exhaustion to regular kindergarten-teacher tired.

The point of all of my rambling about those first two weeks is that I was *not* thinking about germ-killing during that time. I was in survival mode. I didn't scrub my house during those two weeks. I didn't take a shower when I got home from school. I want to say I washed my hands before

I grabbed Itty Bear when I got home each day, but I wouldn't stake my life on it. So, it was no surprise what happened next.

Myles was just shy of five months old. And he started running a fever.

We took him to his doctor. The routine was the same every time. She checked him out, listened to his chest, and tested him for flu and strep. Already, I was expecting the negative test results. And we got them. I wasn't surprised this time. I (and Cash and Max) had been carrying germs home by the gazillions. I would be surprised if he *hadn't* caught something.

She diagnosed him with a virus. And this is when the crushing guilt started settling in.

IT'S ALL MY FAULT

My little baby is laying listlessly on my bare skin. I was hoping he would nurse—he's so small and he's been vomiting and I am praying for God to heal him and help him drink and cool off and recover. This *virus* is hitting him harder than the last two. I put cool, wet wash clothes on his back and under his neck and arms. He vomits up the Tylenol so this is the best I can do.

Why didn't I keep him away from everyone? Why didn't I do a better job cleaning and disinfecting our home? I should have washed my hands more often. I should have made everyone around him wash their hands more often. *I should have quit my job and stayed home with him like I did my other kids when they were babies.*

I don't want to make generalizations about other people, but as I am a part of this particular population I am going to take the liberty to do so: there is no feeling of guilt like the guilt felt by a mother of a sick child. Maybe I'm wrong and most other mothers don't feel that it is their responsibility--their fault--when their child gets sick. After all, in most cases (caveat: those where there is a loving family who tries to do the best for their children) it is not anyone's fault when a child gets sick. There are always exceptions to the rule. But in general, I truly believe that many mothers feel like they did something wrong, or at the very least that there was something they could've done better when their child is very sick. That feeling is absolutely the worst.

To compound my self-condemnation, during this particular episode I had legitimate reasons to blame myself. I really *should* have done better at disinfecting the house and making everyone wash their hands. Being tired and busy was my excuse, but I should've done it anyway.

However, I also had intrusive thoughts that may *not* have been justified: maybe if I had eaten more fruit or more meat while I was pregnant, his immunity would be better. And what about my diet now? I feel like I eat pretty nutritiously (I'd been nursing since Cash was born so I tried to make healthy choices) but I could do better. Is what I eat, or what I don't eat, making my milk inferior? Is that why he was sick? And then there was this one: Am I too old? If I was a younger mother, maybe he wouldn't be getting sick now. The "geriatric pregnancy" diagnosis kept recurring on the playlist of *my failures as a mother*.

In reality, I know in my heart that some of those things weren't my fault. God made Myles exactly when he wanted and how he wanted. He also blessed me with a healthy pregnancy and birth, despite my age—things like that don't hinder God (remember Abraham and Sarah?). However, knowing something and believing it are two different things. With a hot, miserable baby lying in my arms, I felt like the absolute worst mother in the world.

After three days and nights of Myles laying lifelessly on me, he was still running a temperature of 103.9. He wasn't vomiting but he also wasn't eating much. The lymph nodes in his neck felt like two smooth stones implanted under the surface of his skin. We decided to take him back to the doctor. Maybe by this time one of the tests would be positive so we could see what we were dealing with. Surely this wasn't really just a virus. He might need an antibiotic. This was too long for a five-month-old to have an unexplained fever.

When I called to make the appointment they said, *Of course. Bring him right in.* The receptionist sounded concerned when I told her how hot he still was. The high fever combined with not knowing *why* he was sick was very concerning. I took him in, they checked him out and ran tests. And the tests were negative. Again.

We were still seeing the nurse practitioner at this point, and each visit was starting to seem like a replication of the one before. She would greet Myles with care and concern, check him out thoroughly, and find nothing (aside from a fever and swollen lymph nodes) wrong. On our way out the door she would tease, *I don't want to see you for a while*, and tell us to call or come back if his symptoms got worse (*worse?!?)* or his fever didn't go away in a couple of days. This visit was no different, other than being a follow-up because his fever had lasted for so long.

As I carried him out of the office dressed only in his diaper, I threw my favorite olive-colored bamboo swaddle over him to block the sun from his eyes. I was praying as I secured him in his car seat, hoping the heat would soon leave his little body.

Around 2:00 a.m. the next morning, it did. And then he slept. And slept. And slept some more.

When he woke up, our wild, crazy, *healthy* baby was back. And we were thrilled to see him!

When Myles was sick, I would hold him. When I needed a break (I had to pee occasionally), Shawn would nestle him on his shoulder. When Myles was very hot he wouldn't nurse, but he still seemed most comfortable laying on me with the nipple close, so I held him 99 percent of the time. Shawn would check on us through the day and night, bringing the baby his Tylenol or getting me a drink, but he was content to let me hold him.

With Myles in my arms, I could sleep a little. You know how when they put a newborn baby on their mother's chest and they start nursing it makes mother and baby relax? Their breathing and heart rates sync up and slow down. That's what it was like for us when Myles was sick. If I was holding him, we could both relax a little.

We soon had a routine, although it wasn't something we had planned. I would hold Myles, nursing him when he wasn't so hot that he couldn't eat. Shawn took care of Cash and Max and brought us what we needed.

Myles seemed to already have a routine as well. He would usually feel a little rough the day before he got hot, start running a fever during the night, and vomit when his fever peaked. After a few days, the fever would break in the middle of the night. He would sleep for hours the next day. When he woke up, he was back to our crazy little wild boy. Over the following months, this pattern would only continue to grow more familiar.

Now we were in the *after* part of his routine. He had slept half the day and woke up feeling great. When he was running a fever it was like being in a deep, dark hole and not being able to see a way out. When your child is sick—I mean really, really sick—nothing else matters. Not your car, not your job, not your house. *Please, God, please get Myles through the night and make him better.* It's not something you get used to. Not really. When we were in the depths of it, it was dark.

Now, he was happy and healthy, and I was convinced he would never get sick like that again. Our wild boy was back to stay.

Your mind has a funny way of making you feel like *right now* is the only time that exists. Right now, watching our healthy baby boy, I could not imagine a time when he would be sick again.

Thank you, God, for each precious day. For every moment, every smile, every breath.

Life moved on. My sweet group of kindergartners were learning and growing and had quickly become accustomed to the day-to-day experiences of being in school. The boys had fallen into their own routines. Things felt *settled. Calm.* While this would have seemed boring to a much, *much*, younger me, it felt extraordinary to me now.

I hate to say it was the calm before the storm, but *it was the calm before the storm...*

We made it till the middle of September.

RERUNS

Myles had been a little different the day before—not really sick, but just not his normal, bubbly self. Around two a.m. I rolled over and opened one eye to peak at Itty. Something about the way he looked, even in the dark, made me reach out and touch him. His skin was on fire.

I bounced out of bed and grabbed the thermometer. 104.2.

Shaaawwnnn! Wake up!

Could my husband magically make the baby's temperature go down? No. But I was scared and worried and I felt just a tiny bit better knowing that he was awake and scared with me.

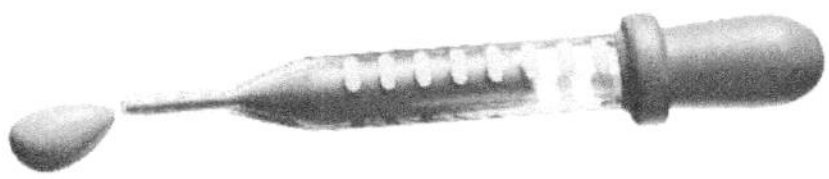

Giving medicine always created a dilemma for me when Myles got hot at night. Did I risk waking him to give him a dose of Motrin or Tylenol or should I let him sleep? When his temp was *this* high, I didn't really have much of a choice.

I put the syringe into his mouth, dispensing the liquid drop by drop until it was all gone (aiming for his cheek so his tongue wouldn't push it out—I'd learned all the tricks by now). It's amazing how long it seems to take to get that little bitty amount of medicine down when you're in such a hurry to get it done, but you only dare push out one drop at a time. But, finally, I squeezed out the last drop...

Blechhhhhh!!

Every single drop of Motrin that I had just painstakingly gotten into the baby shot out faster than Max can scale a door frame (and he can scale a door frame really, *really* fast). It didn't take us many times to realize that it was almost impossible to give Myles liquid medication when he was running a high fever. It would inevitably come right back up. We soon learned that we could use acetaminophen suppositories. But neither ibuprofen nor acetaminophen usually helped much anyway, so we only did that when he was at his hottest and felt like we *had* to try something.

As soon as it was daylight we started trying to get an appointment to take him in and get him seen by a doctor. For whatever reason, we couldn't get him in with his normal NP, so I took him to our local urgent care. They had opened the previous year and had short wait times (which was a big plus), but the downside was you never knew what doctor was going to be working when you showed up. That day, the doctor was friendly and did a thorough check up. They did the normal tests (all negatives, of course), but they didn't try to guess at a diagnosis. After the experience of being prescribed antibiotics when he didn't really need them (at the ER), I was relieved that they didn't take a chance at misdiagnosing him just to give me some kind of answer. No answer was better than a wrong one.

We were sent home with instructions to watch him, treat his fever, and come back if his symptoms worsened. Instructions we had memorized several visits ago.

Three days later, we were back. Myles had developed a cough. This was a new symptom! With this new symptom (and an x-ray), we got an actual diagnosis: pneumonia. Definitely not something to be happy about, but at least we knew what was making him sick this time. With a nebulizer (aka: breathing machine) and a prescription for albuterol we were on our way. After a few more days of fever, breathing treatments, and sleepless nights, Itty bear was back to being our wild, crazy boy.

For a few days. Less than a week. Then we were back at the urgent care center with our baby boy, who was running over 103° fever. This time, when they did the swabs to test for all the things, one came back positive.

He had the flu. Flu A to be specific. When he was well, it was hard for me to imagine him being sick again. Now that he was sick (and had been for days and days—with a couple of short breaks in between) it was hard to imagine a time when he was healthy, laughing, and playing. Right then, he was so weak and so warm. His little body felt like a heating pad as he lay against me.

It didn't take long before I became a human thermometer—I could accurately tell Myles' temperature within about a half degree. I was still compulsively checking it with a real thermometer, but mostly just so I had something new to report when family members called to check on him. If I could say *his temp's gone down to 103.4°* (when an hour ago it had been 103.8°) at least I had some good news to report. I guess I was doing it for myself, too. It was like an obsession. I had to know what his temperature was, and even when I got good at guessing it, I would check myself.

After a few days he got better, but this time was different than the others. Before, he would be deathly sick then the fever would break and he would sleep half a day. When he woke up he was instantly himself again. This time,

(I supposed because he had the flu) he had a hard time bouncing back. As a mother, I could already tell the difference between the fever episodes he was having and the illnesses he had in between the episodes. Back then, I didn't realize that they were *fever episodes,* but I knew there was something different about the way he was sick.

Over the next five months, Myles ran a temperature (a very *high* temperature) ten times. Each of those times, his temperature remained high for anywhere from three to six days. Of those ten occurrences, Myles was diagnosed with Flu A one time and RSV another. We were to assume the others were likely viruses.

It was during this time a pattern emerged.

Other than the Flu and RSV episodes, Myles' fevers were becoming regular. The same number of days would pass between them. The pattern would change occasionally, but it was regular enough that it was odd. Suspicious. He would get a fever every two weeks. After a while it would be every three weeks. Then back to two. But it would stay in the pattern for a while before changing.

We noticed something else, too. When he was getting fevers that were close together, the episodes weren't as severe. If the spacing was farther apart (four weeks, for example), they were terrible.

Now, when I said earlier that they weren't *as severe*, I meant that instead of 105° he might top out at 103°-104°, and instead of lasting five or six days they would last for three. They were still scary and awful, but they just weren't as bad as the others.

We were so scared for our baby. At this point, he was almost a one-year-old. Things were not getting better. We had no answers. I hated taking him to the doctor, and often felt like they thought I was either a hypochondriac or just a bad mother. Heck, *I* thought I was a bad mother. Why was I letting my baby get sick? Over and over and over?

I loved his nurse practitioner, but we weren't getting any answers. At that time, we were primarily taking Myles to her. We would take him to Urgent Care or the emergency room if he got really sick on a weekend or other day she wasn't in the office, but she was our first choice. My family complained to me that she wasn't doing anything. I felt like she was trying, but Shawn and I were also getting frustrated with the lack of a diagnosis. If these were really "just viruses" was his immune system compromised? Why was his little body reacting so strongly to a virus? I had four children before him and had never dealt with such high fevers before. I'd worked in a daycare nursery, had babysit since I was 12, and taught elementary school—I had a lot of experience with sick kids. Children did not have 105° fevers for run of the mill viruses. It just didn't happen. They didn't have 105° fevers for anything that I had ever dealt with.

Once I was taking care of a baby in the nursery who was fine when he laid down for a nap, then minutes later I looked in on him and he looked *different*. Mottled. I touched him and he was on fire. His temperature was 103°. I called his mom, *Get here, now!* Scared the life out of her.

Now *my* baby had temperatures that high--and higher--and it was a regular part of our lives. We were just supposed to move on and accept it. Act like it was normal. That's what the doctors were doing. *Looks like he's got another virus.*

Habituation: decrease in responsiveness upon repeated exposure to a stimulus (Merriam-Webster, 2024)

To a point, we did get used to it. It is human nature to acclimate to your new circumstances, no matter how awful they may be. This process is what allows humans to become survivors. It also contributes to people staying in bad relationships or working at a job they aren't meant to do, for years and years. In certain situations, it is perfectly fine—good, even—to become acclimated to something.

Other times, you need to stop and say *this is not normal. And I am going to be the one to change it.*

THE ROAD NOT TAKEN

Something was wrong, and I would keep pushing until someone found out what it was. So near his first birthday, we started taking Myles to a different doctor.

This is one of those times you've got to use your head more than your heart. I loved the NP we'd been seeing. She was kind and good and really seemed to care about my boy. But if your child's life and health are at stake and you aren't getting answers (not helpful ones, anyway), maybe it's time to get a second opinion. A fresh set of eyes never hurts. Can you imagine a homicide with only one investigator on the case? This was a mystery, and I was the armchair detective, but we needed a professional in the mix.

Cash and Max had been going to an office in an adjoining town. I hesitated to move Myles to that practice because I didn't like driving with him when he was hot. Even though it was less than a half hour away, I was afraid he would have a seizure or vomit and get choked, or something else would happen. I wouldn't see it or be able to do anything to help him because I was driving. To be fair, I had those same irrational thoughts/fears even when my babies weren't sick—I wanted them in my sight and within my grasp at all times (admitted helicopter mom)—but those thoughts weren't so irrational when he was in that condition. Regardless, we had to try another doctor, so I would make the short drive to the next town.

Keep taking the same road and you'll always end up at the same place. We were changing directions.

IT'S THE END OF THE WORLD AS WE KNOW IT

And then...a roadblock.

And this was a doozy.

Toward the end of Myles' first year of life, the world turned upside down. (Anytime I hear those words, I have to sing it in my head as I read: *the wooorld turned upside dowwwn* from my favorite musical, *Hamilton*. I know...real original, right? If you ask 100 people, 99 of them would probably say *Hamilton* was their favorite, too.)

Reports of a strange, deadly new virus were brewing.

Coronavirus

COVID-19

SARS-CoV-2

Everyone was watching China grapple with this illness that was quickly spreading and taking lives. Fortunately, we lived in America so we had nothing to worry about, but it was still something to make small talk about with coworkers and friends. And the conspiracy theories that came with it...wow.

But soon it wasn't just a fun conversation starter—it was real and it was in the U.S.

This book is not about COVID-19, but you can't live through a pandemic without it affecting you and your story. It touched everyone. Some lost their lives or their family members, while others lost their jobs or were otherwise impacted financially...but *everyone* was affected.

Because we had a child who was getting sick every two to four weeks, our lives were very much impacted by the pandemic. However, the doctor visits and lockdowns weren't the only consequences COVID had on our family.

Shawn's mother had been a life-long smoker and liked to collect *things* for many years. As my mother-in-law, it was easy for me to judge her for her life choices. I've learned, through the years, you don't know why someone does what they do until you walk in their shoes—and that's impossible. You don't know what they are going through, and you certainly don't know what they have been through. Recently, I read something that said that you only see a small fraction of what people are actually dealing with. Think about it—when *you* are struggling, do you let everyone see it?

Shawn's mom went through things I could not imagine, and I wouldn't want to trade places with her for all the money in Fort Knox. Who knows what I would have done in her place? I know she loved her kids. And she loved her grandkids. She would always pick up things at the local Goodwill or at a yard sale for my boys. (It drove me crazy.) It made them happy. They knew their Nana loved them, and that's what's important.

There were reports of COVID 19 in our little town around Myles' first birthday. Shawn's mom was sick, and we finally talked her into going to the local emergency room to get checked out. At this time, everyone was on lockdown so the only contact we had with her was through phone calls and saying hello from outside the door when we dropped off food. We were especially worried about her health because of the smoking, and the state of the house...well. We had begged her to let us help clean it out—she was having none of that. Even before this her breathing was labored. But now, she had to catch her breath between words.

So, she drove herself to the local ER.

We were shocked when she called to say she had returned home from the hospital. They didn't admit her! We weren't sure if they even tested her (for COVID). It was very hard to get a test at that time. Half the country was still pretending that COVID didn't exist.

About two weeks before his mom was sick, Shawn was sick. I feel like I've probably seen him at his worst, but I had never seen him in a condition like the one he was in. He was *sick.* And not the normal "man-sick," but knocking on death's door-sick. I wanted him to go to the doctor, but he couldn't sit up. I definitely should have called an ambulance, but Shawn has always been very resistant to getting medical attention and as sick as he was, he was able to protest just enough that I didn't call for help. He had a horrible cough and was having fever dreams. He would talk in his sleep as he tossed and turned. I prayed hard and played nurse, bringing him medicine and cool washcloths, and forcing him to drink until he was well. It was a scary time, and I am certain he had COVID, though he was never tested.

As soon as he was well, I was sick. I had the same symptoms, but I was never in the shape he was in. I stayed conscious, but I was weak and coughing. For the first time in my life, I felt like I couldn't get enough oxygen.

Unlike my very stubborn husband, I *did* go to the local urgent care center. I didn't request a COVID test—I just wanted them to tell me what was wrong with me and give me something to make it go away. Strangely, I was immediately met with hostility.

Are you here looking for a COVID test? The doctor's voice was angry as soon as she came to my car window.

No, I responded. *I just want to see a doctor. I've been running a fever for two days now so I thought I should get checked out. It's kind of hard to breathe.*

Well, huffed the doctor, *we aren't just going to test you because you have a temperature and think you can't breathe as well as you'd like.* (Again, **I never asked for a test**, or even mentioned coronavirus.) *There haven't been any cases around here so there's no way you have COVID.*

So, here's the little problem with that: the local radio station had announced three cases in our small town just days before. They could wish it away all they wanted, but that wasn't stopping it. And this was a medical *professional* pretending it wasn't here.

I don't know if I had COVID, and I can't say for a fact that Shawn had COVID the week before. After the belligerent reception I received from the doctor, there was no way I was going to tell her about my suspicions about him. I will always believe that he did, but I'll never know for sure.

Just like we'll never know for sure about his mom.

After she was sent home from the emergency department, Shawn called his brother so they could figure out what, if anything, they could do. I had complained and preached about getting his mom out of her house and into a safe place (or at the very least just cleaning out *her* place) for so long. I kept chiming in on Shawn's phone conversation with his brother, so he finally just said, *Here,* and thrust the phone into my hand. His brother and I had a great discussion. Things had to change. We made a plan to work together and clean out her house just as soon as she got over this current illness. She might protest, (Who am I kidding? She would throw a fit.) but we were all on the same page and we would work together to make things better for her.

It's hard when your parents get older. I still remember when my mom and her sisters had to take the car keys from my grandpa. He was strong and good, the person we all looked up to. He was the leader of our family. It was unnerving to see *them* taking care of *him.* It was unnatural. But even then, as a child, I knew it had to be done to protect him and keep other travelers safe. This, too, would be uncomfortable and hard, but we knew it had to be done.

And even though it was going to be difficult, there was a silver lining. We were finally going to make things better for her! I actually got a rush when I thought about that part of it. This had been a long time coming and it was kind of like doing an extreme home makeover. It reminded me of the day she let me clean up her kitchen a little bit—such a small task, but the emotional payoff was enormous. Decluttering was like a drug, with no negative side effects.

I went to bed that night with a sense of peace and accomplishment. We hadn't done the hard part yet, but everyone was on board and we had a plan.

Two days later it was Easter morning. Such a strange Easter. COVID made everything feel different. We should be going to church, then having lunch at my mom's and an egg hunt with our family. Instead, we were sitting on the kitchen floor watching the boys look through their Easter baskets. I was recording it with my phone so we could share it with our families. Then the phone started ringing. I didn't want to stop recording the kids so I just sent the call to voicemail. After it stopped, it immediately started ringing again. Begrudgingly, I looked to see who was calling. It was

Shawn's mom, so I answered. She asked for him. After speaking with her for a minute, he hung up.

I have to go to my mom's.

Is something wrong? I asked. I knew she was sick but she had seemed a little better the day before so I thought she was on the road to recovery.

I don't know. But I need to go see.

Shawn was back in fifteen minutes. I could tell how worried he was. He paced around the house mumbling, *It's really bad. It's really bad.* He had left so quickly to check on her that he had forgotten to take his phone, and I realized that's what he was looking for.

She's in bad shape. She wants me to get her a drink at Five Star and she says she's having trouble breathing.

We need to call 911! I insisted as I found his phone (it was *hiding* on the charger) and pushed it into his hand.

I don't know what to do. She doesn't want to go to the hospital! Just let me go take her a drink and I'll see how she is then.

We argued for a second before he said, *Okay! Just call them!* Then he was out the door as I quickly dialed 911.

Five minutes later, my phone rang.

My mom's dead!!!

The ambulance had gotten to her at the same time Shawn had. She had been talking to him minutes before. She was gone before he could get back.

Shawn struggled, and I do mean *struggled* with losing his mom. He felt guilty for not staying with her (even though she had sent him away to get her a drink). He felt guilty that he hadn't done more for her (even though he did everything he could to help her from the time he was a small child). If she needed something, he dropped everything else and did it. He felt so guilty for things he shouldn't have felt guilty about. It is strange how emotions work sometimes.

P- WHAT?

Life moved on, as it does. We were seeing the new doctor frequently, because the episodes were relentless. Even so, we had gotten to the point where we didn't take him to see the doctor *every* time he got a fever. Almost all the visits went the same. They ran tests, I would say something like, *Don't you think something weird is going on?* Then we would go home with a sick baby, unanswered questions, and instructions to watch him and treat his fever. *Watch him and treat his fever*. What good was that doing?

We took him to the doctor when his fever was so high it scared us, which was about every other episode. Even if we had been completely comfortable with the high fevers, we would still take him at least every other time with the hopes that one of those visits would be different. Eventually someone had to say, *This isn't normal, let's find out what's wrong*. And finally, someone did.

I've been thinking a lot about this. About Myles. I wonder if he could have a fever disorder.

Myles' pediatrician had just examined him, and I was ready for the, *Keep an eye on him. Treat his fever and call if you need us*, so her words caught me off-guard.

At the mention of a potential diagnosis, my heart sped up and I leaned forward in my chair, fully invested in what Dr. Avery was saying.

There's someone who works in this office...her son has PFAPA.

P- what? I questioned Myles' doctor.

PFAPA. It's a fever disorder.

She began telling me what she knew about the disorder. Everything about Myles' patterns of fevers and the symptoms that came with them feel right into place. She said she only knew about the disorder because one of her coworkers had a son who was diagnosed with it a few years earlier.

PFAPA stands for periodic fever, aphthous stomatitis, pharyngitis, adenitis. It's a syndrome that causes children to have periodic fevers. Never heard of it? I hadn't either, and, unfortunately, neither have many doctors.

Again, this "PFAPA" was totally new to me, but I now had the most wonderful thing: hope. Someone had finally acknowledged that Myles had something going on. Not only that, but she had even given me a possible diagnosis!

My head was spinning, and I drove home on autopilot as thoughts cascaded through my mind. As soon as I walked in the door, I told Shawn we finally might have an answer. I told everyone who asked about Myles, *We think we know what's wrong! PFAPA!* I received confused looks, but I was happy to explain what I had learned.

Out of 10,000 children only two—2.3 actually, but where they found that third of a kid we'll never know–will have PFAPA (Wang et al., 2021).

I can't believe it took the doctors this long to figure it out!

Yeah... That didn't make sense to us either. His symptoms are identical to the PFAPA symptoms.

What are they doing to stop it?

Well, nothing yet. But I'm looking into it. As soon as he sees the specialist we'll know more. Hopefully we get a treatment plan worked out before his next episode.

Wouldn't that be wonderful! Well, we're praying for your family and for little Myles. Please keep us updated.

I immediately started googling this rare syndrome to learn all I could about it. I dove into the research. It was amazing how Myles' symptoms paralleled the description of the disorder. The patterns finally made sense! We were going to get our baby (well, actually *toddler*, now) diagnosed and make him well!

But, as almost everything goes in the bureaucratic medical system, it would not be that easy. And coronavirus made it that much harder.

COVID made the whole world slow down. Now, if you're an introvert (like me) the lockdown part of COVID was an amazing perk to an otherwise horrific time in history. I loved being at home with my family. Taking hour-long baths then curling up with a warm blanket (and a kid or two) to browse Amazon or read a book? Phenomenal! Spending as much time as I wanted helping the boys with their schoolwork? Outstanding! But, I also had an undiagnosed sick child. I needed to find out what was wrong with him so we could stop it. That was pretty hard to do when you could barely leave the house.

The other way coronavirus affected us (or I should say *one* of the other ways, but this was a big one) was that it added another uncomfortable test that Myles had to go through every single time we took him to the doctor's office. On the news, we would frequently hear about adults who whined and complained about having to take one COVID test before they did things like fly on an airplane or visit a different state or country. I understood that it caused an inconvenience to some people, but as the mom of a baby who had to get it done frequently, I wanted to shout, *Be thankful you don't have to put your child through this when he already feels bad! You are adults and you're choosing to travel! He's a baby, and he doesn't have a choice about getting sick.* Of course, I didn't do that. But I wanted to.

Myles was already getting strep and flu tests, and often blood work, and now he had this other test to add: getting another Q-Tip shoved up his nose. To put it bluntly, it sucked.

Not only that, for months he would have to quarantine every time he had a fever. This part was the hardest on our family members. They were pretty attached to Itty, who was the baby of the family. Going a week or longer (one time it was a whole month) with only visits on FaceTime or through the window, was heartbreaking. I still remember holding him up to our glass storm door to talk to Grandma and Aunt MeMe. He didn't understand why they weren't taking him when he reached his little arms out. I remember several times watching my mom walk away in tears after visiting with the boys through the glass door.

If we had known for sure that Myles didn't have COVID, we probably wouldn't have worried as much about keeping the people who were closest to us away from him (consequently away from us as well). We couldn't know for sure. And we'd already lost one grandparent to COVID. So we took precautions.

With the pandemic making things harder on Myles, harder on us, and harder on our extended family who were missing out on milestones (he turned one in the spring of 2020) we were more determined than ever to find out what was causing Myles to be sick. It felt like the old adage, though: one step forward and two steps back (another phrase I can't say without singing it in my head). We had this possible diagnosis, but it was harder than ever to get appointments of any kind—particularly appointments with specialists. Eventually, though, we did get an appointment. Myles' doctor (the one who suggested PFAPA) decided to send him to a specialist at the University of Kentucky. It was a doctor with the Infectious Disease department. This was great! At that time, my daughter was living in Lexington and attending UK. She was also taking medical classes and had observed in the offices where we would be going for this appointment. I felt good knowing there was a connection.

During the weeks leading up to Myles' first visit with the Infectious Disease doctor, I was experiencing a whirlwind of emotions. I was so full of hope, so sure that this one visit would change our lives. It *had* to be PFAPA. While that's not a curable disease, it *is* treatable. It also sort of resolves itself as the child ages. In most cases, the fever episodes cease by adulthood. The length between fevers spread until the episodes stop.

Hope.

But for now, Myles' episodes were full speed ahead with no end in sight. We'd get a little time to breathe, catch up on sleep...then, boom! 104°... 105°.... *Is it time for his appointment yet?*

It was hard to stay positive when he was still getting so sick. And since we *knew* what he had, why did it take weeks and weeks to get him treated? Before all this, I could not imagine letting a child be this sick for days (let alone weeks or months) when there was medicine that could stop it. My idyllic view of the American medical system had been fractured, but in the coming months, it would be completely shattered.

At the worst the fevers were two weeks apart. At the very best: five. We were at the worst while we waited for his visit with the doctor who was going to cure him (well, not *cure*, but diagnose and treat him). Fortunately, he felt normal in between episodes so he had days of feeling good, but the days when he wasn't feeling good were *so* bad. Getting used to seeing my little boy lay in my arms with a high fever (and all that comes with it—the sore throat, the stomach pain, the vomiting) is something I will never get used to. Every time, when he was well, I would forget how bad it was.

There is no pain like watching your child suffer. I think my brain let me forget a little in between episodes. While he was restlessly sleeping I would cry, *I'm so sorry. I'm so sorry. I'm so sorry.* Thinking about it now takes me back to that moment in time. I feel his fevered little body sweltering on my chest, the faintly sweet smell of sweat mixed with *baby*. I'm watching his little belly rise and fall as the middle of his tiny chest beats in and out so quickly. His eyelids parted slightly so it was hard to tell if he was fully asleep or conscious. He would sleep so much when he was sick, but never fully rest. Most unnerving to me was when his little body would start twitching. Was *this* a seizure? This would go on for days.

Then it would stop.

LIE TO ME

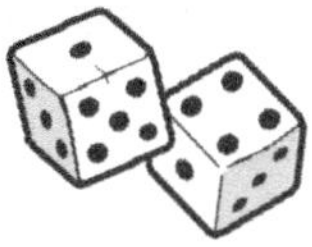

We were fairly confident that Itty had a fever disorder, even though he had not been diagnosed. During the period between *knowing* what it probably was and having an actual diagnosis was frustrating in its own way. We knew there was not a lot a regular doctor could do for him until he was diagnosed and had a treatment plan. That's why we didn't go to the doctor every time he had a fever. However, just like any child, he could still get COVID or the flu or any other illness. His body also didn't respond to fever-reducers like Tylenol and Motrin the same way most people's did. Sometimes they would help his fever go down a little, sometimes they wouldn't do anything. So, when Myles' fever hit 105 and then kept climbing towards 106, we rushed him to the hospital a few towns over (the closest one with a pediatric wing).

Even though we were fairly certain this was a normal episode, we always got nervous when his fever was this high. If something did happen, I wanted Myles to be in the care of professionals. Would they be knowledgeable, caring professionals? We didn't know, but we were going to roll the dice.

We checked into the ER and the nurse didn't hide her concern as she quickly took us right back to a cubicle. There's an overwhelming trend when you take your very sick child to the doctor then they are suddenly much better when they get there, or at the very least their *high* temperature has decreased significantly by the time a nurse runs the wand across their forehead. (I remember my mother telling me, *You always acted like you were fine when we got to the doctor.)* It can make moms look—or at least *feel*—crazy. I *wish* that would have happened. His fever read 105.8°.

The doctor came in quickly. I answered questions while they tried to get him to drink Motrin (which he proceeded to vomit all over the nurse and I. Me: *He can't drink medicine when he's this hot.* Her: *It'll be fine.*). They ran bloodwork, did all the nose and mouth swabs, and I explained that we were seeing a specialist soon to confirm that he had a fever disorder.

The biggest problem with going to the ER, in my humble opinion, is that you never know what kind of doctor you are going to get. Growing up in a small town, my family and I have debated/discussed which local hospital is better multiple times, but it all really comes down to the doctor on call. For example, several years ago in the county

I grew up in, a man was rushed to the hospital. The doctor who was working in the ER that night examined him. The man was dying. In fact, he was going to go so quickly that there was no need to call a helicopter to fly him out.

You need to say your goodbyes, the doctor told the family.

Calls were made. Prayer wheels were started. The family was devastated. This was the beloved patriarch of their family. They said their goodbyes. Except one person didn't. She threw a fit.

She said, *You will transfer him right now. I want a second opinion!*

And guess what? The ER doctor on call had been completely wrong. The *dying* man was up and walking around just a couple of days later, and I believe he is still alive today. True story. It matters who is on call.

Well, that night we had a doctor who was not only unfamiliar with fever disorders (as I was a few weeks before this, but ***I am not a doctor***), but he was also determined to find a cause for Itty's high fever, then get us out the door.

Has he been coughing?

No.

Been around someone with COVID?

Not that I'm aware of. We keep him pretty isolated.

Runny nose?

No.

I won't bore you with the rest, but he had a lot of questions.

I explained again about fever disorders.

Let's get a chest x-ray.

Okay.

Within two hours we were on our way home--with a diagnosis of pneumonia. Did he have symptoms of pneumonia? Well, he had a fever. That was his only symptom (unless you count the vomiting that was triggered by being hot and having to drink Motrin.) Myles' fever was under 104, so we were back in familiar territory. We had instructions to follow up with his pediatrician the next day, so we did. Amazingly, the pneumonia had gone away—in less than 24 hours.

I did not count all of the episodes Myles had before it was finally time for his appointment with the specialist, but I know it was a lot. It was more fevers than many people have in a lifetime. He was a year and a half old. It was finally the big day.

APPOINTMENT DAY

...and I go a little off the rails. Sorry.

The day we had all been waiting for had finally arrived. While I did not have the exact number of fever episodes Myles had had at the ready, I had been tracking them ever since we knew he might have PFAPA and I had the records from the times I had taken him to the doctor. I knew that his pediatrician had sent enough information in the referral to let the specialist know that he was a very sick baby, and that his fevers were episodic, but I also took the records I had to impress upon her just how significant his illness was. I had done my research, so I knew that it was an unmistakable case of PFAPA. While there were other fever disorders I had learned about through my deep dive into the condition, his symptoms aligned perfectly with this disorder, and the others had disqualifying symptoms and/or cultural background requirements.

On the big day, we all got up early and got ready for the almost two-hour trip to Lexington. Shawn, Myles, and I would be going alone, so we dropped Cash and Max off at Aunt MeMe's for the day. Not only was this right in the midst of the pandemic (so we wanted to limit their exposure), but all of our boys got motion sickness pretty easily, so we kept car rides to a minimum. Itty slept almost the whole way to Lexington. As crazy as it sounds, it was almost like being on a date (if you could put the unpleasant reason for our drive out of mind for a moment). We listened to music for a while, but mostly we just talked. It was nice. The baby was currently between episodes, so life was good. We had lots to be thankful for, and in a few hours' time we could add one more thing: Myles would have a diagnosis and a treatment plan in place. This nightmare would soon be over.

About ten minutes before we arrived at the clinic Myles woke up. About five minutes after that, he vomited all over himself and his car seat. Hey, we were just happy it happened then and not halfway through our trip, in a place where we couldn't pull over for miles. As it was, I just climbed over the seat and cleaned him up the best I could. Being a mother is amazing. You do things you never expected. Like cleaning up vomit while driving past the castle of Versailles. (That's ver-SAYLZ, by the way...and if you've never heard of the Kentucky Castle you should really check it out.)

Just moments later, we were pulling into the parking garage. I had been keyed up all day, wired like a teenage girl in a room with Austin Butler. When Shawn turned off the ignition, it was like my body went into fight or flight. My stomach dropped. My heart palpitated. I know it sounds crazy, but I had thought about this appointment since our pediatrician said *PFAPA.* I dreamt about this appointment in the minutes I slept between waking to make sure Myles wasn't hotter or jerking too much. This was not just any appointment to me. It was the one that would change our lives.

We put on our masks and walked in. Myles did really well with wearing his mask. We had some tiny ones made that fit him comfortably, and he had gotten used to them. We all went through the temperature checks and pandemic questions before we were allowed to into the lobby. Such an odd snapshot in time. Looking back, those days seem more like an apocalyptic fiction than reality. Regardless, we went through all the necessary procedures and got checked in. I noticed the sign *Only one parent may go back with the patient,* but I asked the nurse if we could both go since it was his first visit.

Let me check with the doctor, replied the receptionist.

A few minutes later, a nurse called out *Myles Hare* and I jumped up and headed her way. She indicated toward Shawn, *Dad can come on back, too.* I breathed a silent prayer as we headed back. Another small step towards our answers.

The visit was not what I expected. UK is a teaching hospital. That has various implications. It can be a very good thing because *teaching* is directly linked with *learning*. As a teacher, I would put it like this: when I graduated with my degree in P-5 education, I was taught how to teach reading. They taught me based on the current information they had on best practices. In recent years, I have been continuing my education. The classes I have been taking include the newest research. We now know more about the brain and how to engage it to help children learn better, easier, and faster. We use the science of reading to help all kids learn better. If I had decided that I was not going to further my education after obtaining my degree, I would not have learned these better practices and I would have continued teaching the same way I was taught fifteen years ago. The biggest implication of that is that all of my present and future students would suffer because I was not teaching them using the most current and research-proven methods. They might learn, but maybe not as quickly or as in-depth as they would have if I had done my part to stay abreast of the most up-to-date information. I might even miss that a child had a learning disability or need of some kind because I had not been educated on the signs to look for.

That's the positive part of being a teaching hospital (at least, from a patient perspective). The doctors, nurses, interns, and residents are all involved in researching the latest data. That's a *really* big positive. Especially when your child could have a rare disease.

Even though being up-to-date with the latest research on education is very important, I would say—with no hesitation—knowing the most current information on health issues is significantly more important. Literally, life-or-death important.

To illustrate the side of teaching hospitals which some would consider negative, I think back over two decades ago to when I was pregnant with my first-born daughter, Hailey.

Actually, let's go back a little further, then I promise to wrap back around and tie it all up with a pretty bow. (If you want to skip to the next chapter, it won't hurt my feelings. But you'll miss a pretty wild story.)

There are so many songs about being young...doing crazy things when you were young...being wild and young. I'm going to be very honest here and tell you, I did my fair share.

There is also a saying,

The greatest growth comes from the hardest lesson learned.

When I was in college, I met a boy.

I hate to use the old cliche' ***do you believe in love at first sight?*** But there is really no other accurate way to describe the feeling we got when we met. Here's another one: *it knocked me off my feet*. I was *head over heels* in love with him as soon as I laid eyes on him.

We spent the next seven days together, planning our future, wondering how we had survived the nineteen years before without each other in our lives. (Don't worry—if you're rolling your eyes, laughing because you already know, or have guessed, the ending—I'm right there with you.)

See, there was a timetable on this whole situation: Kane had recently completed boot camp for the United States Navy. The week we met had been his last on the mainland. He was flying out to his first assignment—Hawaii—the next day. An absolute dream come true for most people, a nightmare for two young people in love.

During the *week* we had been together, I got the whole sad story about Kane's home life. I'm not going to say he likes to exaggerate or make things up...

He wanted to get married. ASAP. I was 19 years old, and he was, too. *Hard lessons.*

A few months after he left, he got a 96-hour leave. During leave he was allowed to go off the ship and experience a negligible bit of freedom. Of course, he had rules to follow, and he would have to report back on time. Also, there was a perimeter he had to stay in. Leaving the island was completely off-limits, and breaking any military rules would result in time in the Brig (that's the ship prison—not a fun place, from what I've heard). It also carried the risk of a dishonorable discharge.

But remember, we were young and *in love.* So who cares about consequences? Kane took the first (12 hour) flight to Kentucky. For an $800 plane ticket, and with the risk of jail time, we got two nights and three days together.

When Kane returned to Hawaii, we were even more determined to be together. Of course, the reasonable (I use this word very loosely) option would have been for me to transfer to college in Hawaii and become a military wife so he could finish his Navy career and I could finish my education. We didn't do that. Kane found a way to get discharged from the Navy, and we had a big church wedding a couple of months later.

When Kane and I were happy, we were very, very happy. But when we weren't...well. We were like gasoline poured on a fire. I have never argued with someone like we argued. Eventually I learned not to fight back. Then I learned not to cry, because crying made him very angry. I could internalize it all. Not a healthy option, but I was married (when *everyone* told me, *slow down, you're too young to get married*) so I tried to keep it together. I couldn't prove them right.

I was young and foolish, but I learned from the experience. We all have things we're not proud of, but they teach us and shape us. And I can't regret "Kane," because I have Hailey and Caleb. God can make blessings anytime and anywhere.

Kane had wanted to start a family right away, so he was so happy when he found out I was pregnant after being married for six months. Did things change? Of course not. Not for the better, anyway. Things were never *normal.* We were either crazy in love or setting forest fires. When I was around seven-and-a-half months pregnant, he said he was leaving. He didn't—but it took an emotional toll on me. Not long after that, I went into early labor.

And we are finally back to my point. For those of you who left us for a while, welcome back! I know I went the long (very, very long) way around Robin Hood's barn, but now I'll wrap it all up. When I went into early labor at 32 weeks, I was taken to Vanderbilt University Medical Center. It is known for being the largest research and teaching center in the mid-south region of the U.S. It was amazing. My room was like a hotel room. However, I had no privacy. Kane was upset. My mom was upset. The tension was palpable. I felt like I was in the middle, and there were doctors, nurses, and students coming into my room every five minutes. Literally. *Every five minutes.* Someone would take my blood pressure. Then another person would come in and ask me the same questions I had answered twice already in the last hour. Then someone else would come and take my blood pressure again. At some points, there were at least ten people in my room. I am not exaggerating. I didn't know who to look at, and I didn't know who was in charge.

In addition to all of the aforementioned chaos, I was on two kinds of drugs to halt my labor and they made my heart pound like a Killers song. I would go from heartbroken to hysterically laughing in seconds. It was like being on drugs (which, actually I was--the legal kind), but they were very bad drugs. They were not fun at all. And during all this, I was supposed to be *relaxing* because *stress can cause premature labor*.

Now, imagine that scenario from a child's perspective. At a teaching hospital (or clinic, like the one we were at), you didn't just see the doctor. We were taken back by a nurse who took Myles' vitals, then another nurse came in to do the same thing (blood pressure, oxygen, weight, height). Then a resident came in to talk to us. He asked about a million questions, took notes, then did a physical exam on Myles. As he walked out he said, *Dr. ******* will be right in!* About 30-45 minutes after he left, she came into the room. She was flanked by yet another medical student.

Now, I totally get that a lot of that is necessary, and I mentioned the biggest benefit earlier: being current in research studies. It is also crucial for medical students to practice on real people. But I would be amiss to leave out how this affects a patient who is: number one, a child, and number two, having to make extremely frequent visits to doctors. When you already feel "touched out" and you have to let three or four times as many people put their hands on you, it just makes the experience a little harder.

As a mother, I was supposed to be protecting him. I felt guilty EVERY SINGLE TIME I took Myles to the doctor. He was already miserable and uncomfortable for most of those visits, and I was letting them put things in his nose, gag him with a throat swab (sometimes twice in one visit), and do basically whatever the doctor deemed necessary. I felt helpless. I wanted them to figure out what was wrong, but I was so tired of them doing things to my baby. Hopefully this visit would put an end to that.

As Dr. ******* walked in with her medical student sidekick, she politely introduced herself and the young lady who was with her. She asked questions (the same ones we had answered close to an hour before, but I was happy to answer again). She examined Myles. She asked me if he had ever had mouth sores.

I don't remember him ever having mouth sores, I replied.

This would become a question I heard a lot. And it would become a point of frustration. The thing is, all children who have PFAPA do not have all of the same symptoms. And they definitely don't all have mouth sores. But I'll tell you more about that later.

Dr. ******* talked to Shawn and I while I nursed Itty to calm him down. He was fussy from being handled by strangers yet again. The doctor discussed some tests she wanted to do. Then,

Do you have any questions? she asked.

Well, yes, I had questions. We had waited so long for this visit and she had not mentioned a diagnosis or what she thought could be causing his fevers.

What do you think could be causing his fevers? I asked. I wanted to say, *Do you know how long we have waited to see you? What is wrong with my baby? What are you going to do to fix it?* But I was out of my comfort zone just asking that question so directly, so I politely listened to her answer, nodding in understanding.

Well, we need to do some blood work before I have answers, Dr. ******* responded. *Oh, did they give you the fever chart?* (I nodded, *yes*.) *You'll need to fill that out—just chart his fevers from now on—and when you come back in three months bring it with you.*

Three months? I wanted to scream. My entire body filled with rage, and at the same time I was fighting tears. I didn't want this doctor (or Myles) to see me cry. And I couldn't speak because I didn't know what would come out if I opened my mouth. This baby had been suffering every two to four weeks since he was three months old. She could stop it. I had read so much about PFAPA. I was not a doctor, but I was a *mother*. I was right there with him for every single episode. Though I didn't feel the physical pain, I felt like we went through the episodes together.

I had become obsessed with fever disorders, reading everything I could find. His fevers followed a pattern. He had all the symptoms, and there were treatments that could help. All the hope I had held onto for months vanished in an instant.

The doctor rattled off some instructions about getting a blood draw during his next episode, so I nodded my head as I made sure we had everything packed away in the diaper bag. I was hearing her talk, but my brain had already put her on mute. I'm glad Shawn was there to repeat it to me later when I would be more accepting.

We were silent as we walked down the corridor and exited the building. Shawn got Myles settled in his car seat. I closed my car door, and that's when I fell apart. I cried while Shawn drove. In minutes, Itty was sleeping. That's when I went on a tirade. I (quietly) used language that is not usually a part of my vocabulary. I was so mad. I'm a pretty even-tempered person most of the time, but if I think someone is hurting my kids, I lose it.

I lost it.

The simmering rage I felt as the doctor was brushing off my concerns and turning us away for *a quarter of a year* was now boiling over.

Shawn was probably as upset as I was, but he put his feelings on hold and listened to me express mine. After I got some of the anger and frustration out, he did what he always does: calmed me down. Helped me to see reason. Then, reminded me that being upset was not going to change anything. It would not even speed up this process.

The doctor wanted us to record the next three months of fevers, so I would give her the most detailed fever record she had ever seen.

We had managed this for well over a year. We would make it three more months. I hated that Myles would be miserable through a lot of that time, but we didn't have a choice. Or, at least, we didn't have a *good* choice. What was I going to do? Throw a fit in the doctor's office and demand immediate treatment for my child? The most likely outcome of that scenario would be me being escorted out of the building and the office's refusal to see Myles again, or worse. I guess I could also have taken him back to his pediatrician and asked her to send us to another doctor, but even if she gave us another referral we might have to wait longer than three months just to get in. And who knows if they would tell us anything different? We resigned ourselves to do what the specialist had asked. We would be taking him to get bloodwork the next time his fever skyrocketed (which I could already tell her would be in a week and a half), and we would record his fevers on her *Fever and Symptom Diary.* Just a few more hoops to jump through. It wasn't the life-changing visit I had hoped for, but we were one step closer, right?

A week and a half later...nothing happened! He was cured.

Just kidding.

A week and a half later, he vomited, his temp went up, and we took him for blood work. The results left me floored.

SMOKING GUN

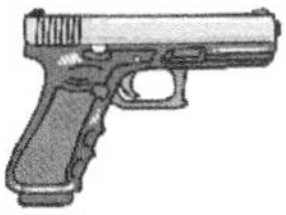

Myles' CRP (C-Reactive Protein) was through the roof. I mean, it was *crazy high*. When you Google *CRP and PFAPA*, the result at the top (from bjbms.org, Kraszewska-Glomba) says *We found CRP levels to be substantially increased during febrile episodes in patients with PFAPA, which is consistent with other studies. In the obtained decision tree, CRP is used as the initial split variable to distinguish viral infections from bacterial infections and PFAPA flares.*

After I recovered from the shock, I realized what I had just been given. Less than two weeks after our visit with Dr. ******* and we had irrefutable proof that he had PFAPA! At the same time I was celebrating the smoking gun we had just been handed, I was hit by the fact that Myles' CRP was extremely high.

Let me explain why that's troubling: when there is inflammation in the body, the liver is triggered to make C-Reactive Protein. The C-Reactive protein binds to damaged tissue, and there are studies showing that it also helps regulate inflammatory processes. The level of CRP that is produced is directly related to the amount of inflammation in the body. Since Myles' CRP levels were extremely elevated, it meant he had a very high amount of inflammation at the time of the test. I always wondered if he was hurting when he had episodes of high fever, and this test gave a very strong indication that he was. As if I wasn't already motivated enough to push for a diagnosis...

I was going to be prepared for the next appointment. I *thought* I was prepared for the first one, but now I felt like I was going to war for my son. The plan was to become as knowledgeable about fever disorders as possible. My goal was to be able to have an intelligent, productive discussion with Dr. *******. Especially if she didn't plan to diagnose him and begin a treatment plan at the next appointment.

Four episodes later (with days in between when you couldn't tell he'd been sick a day in his life), it was time to go back to the Pediatric Infectious Disease unit at UK. Myles had just gotten over a pretty bad episode, and my emotions were raw.

Experiencing your child feel pain or hurt of any kind is hard. Someone once told me that *once you are a mother, you will never be happier than your saddest child.* The words spun around in my head a few times before they made sense. And then, I didn't fully believe them. How could one person's emotional state of being completely depend on that of someone else? Or, as in my case, five someone else's? Once I did become a mother, those words drifted back to me. Now I have a deep understanding of their weight. Four of my children may be happy, healthy, and content. If one of the five (no matter *which* of them it is) has had heartbreak, sickness, physical pain...I am going to hurt with them. They won't understand that—and I don't want them to—until they become a mother or a father. With the deepest love comes the most intense pain.

There is something inside you that changes when you become a parent. It's both physical and intangible. You become forever and completely intertwined with a person who is their own being, yet is also a part of you. Their joy becomes your satisfaction in the same way their distress becomes your agony. Love is the most fulfilling and most painful part of being human. The love we feel for our children may be the closest we could ever get to a glimpse of God's inconceivable and phenomenal love for us.

TAKE TWO

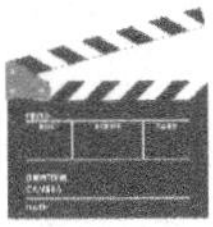

On the ride to the first appointment with Dr. ******* I was giddy—nervous, but excited—because we were going to finally have a treatment plan for Itty. This time I was just nervous. Well...there was also some anger mixed in, but deep down I was just so afraid she would brush us off again that the hostility stayed buried—for now at least.

Monica. Just calm down. Shawn was driving and watching me from the corner of his eye as I was digging through my purse for something of insignificance. The contents spilled out onto the floorboard, rolling under the seat and into cracks where some of them would never be seen again.

I am calm. It's not my fault you can't drive! I snapped. We were currently cruising down a straight road at a smooth fifty-five.

Shawn responded, *Acting all crazy isn't going to change anything.*

I'm not acting crazy! I corrected him.

From the backseat, Cash chimed in, *She's not acting.*

Leave it to Cash to provide a break in the tension that we were all feeling.

After a few minutes, Shawn reminded me, *You have done everything you possibly could to help Myles get better. You probably know more about P-whatever than that doctor does by now. If she doesn't help him, we'll find someone who will, but for right now we are doing all we can.*

I know. I just...

It was so hard to put into words what I was feeling. I knew Shawn was right, but did he feel the overwhelming guilt in the middle of the night when Myles was burning up and limp? He would peek at me through half-closed eyelids and my heart felt like it was being ripped out of my chest.

A few years ago, we had a preacher, Brother Jack, who would come to the little white church on Wednesday nights. He told us about his daughter being sick many, many years ago. Hospitals were much different back then, and parents were not allowed to stay overnight with their children. He reflected on how hard it was to leave her for the night. He and his wife returned as soon as visitors were permitted the following morning. He walked in to see his tiny daughter--*strapped to the bed*--reaching her little arms out and saying, *Help me, daddy*. The way he described feeling on that long-ago day when his child was weak, bound, and quietly asking him to help her is the way I felt every time Myles would look at me when he was sick. I was letting him down. He needed help, and I was failing him. Over and over, I was letting him down. And no one could convince me I wasn't.

Myles and I got out at the door of the office building, and I looped the straps of his Minecraft mask over his ears. Only one parent would be allowed back this time, and since the boys had come with us they were going to hang out in the parking garage with Shawn while Myles and I went in to meet our fate. That's what it felt like, anyway.

We hadn't been in the waiting room long before I heard, *Myles Hare?* I settled Itty on my hip and followed the nurse back, making small talk about the weather like I didn't have a care in the world. It's funny how we can act so polite to strangers even when we are emotionally breaking.

Myles was used to the process by now, but he still didn't like it. He tolerated it much better when he was healthy, like today, but he was also harder to "contain." I'd take him like this any day. Rambunctious and spirited...this is the way a little boy should always be.

Sometimes you could be waiting for hours, but we learned a few tricks over the course of our many office visits:

1. Breastfeeding is a lifesaver—especially when the exam is over and you are trying to listen to the doctor.
2. It's a bad idea to take a lot of toys to scatter, but one or two little things that fit in your purse or diaper bag can help with those long waits both in the room and the waiting area (think drawing boards, fidget toys, or magnets—if your child is old enough to not eat them).
3. YouTube is always a favorite and it's always in your pocket. Yes, the signs say *No Cell Phones*, but if you ask first, most nurses will tell you it's fine to play a video (I just feel like I should thank *The Wiggles* right now) for your baby. The signs are mostly for people who don't know better than to play on their phones—or even take calls—while the doctor is in the room, wasting their precious time. If you keep the volume low and put the phone away when the doc comes in, it usually makes everyone's

job much easier. A child's favorite video is also a great distraction during blood draws or injections. If you want to go the extra mile, purchase some child-safe headphones.

4. The other thing that helped us was counting. Myles was obsessed with numbers and the alphabet by the time he was a year old. When the clip was on his finger and he was wiggling, we would count. When they were drawing blood or doing something else he didn't like, I would say the ABC's and leave out a letter. He would be figuring out the missing letter and correcting me instead of thinking about what was being done to him. Just figure out something they like and use it.

We got through all the check-in stuff. Then an intern came in and asked me all the questions that the doctor would ask again when she came in.

By the time the doctor made it, I was about out of tricks and had offered Myles baboo, so he was hiding in my shirt and drinking contently. Dr. ******* and I discussed the results of the labs, as well as the fever episodes Myles had over the past three months. Although she had the papers in her hand that showed the clockwork-like episodes in black and white, I stressed that point to make sure she was getting it,

He's been really sick. We can look at the calendar and tell within a day when his next fever will be. We've got to do something to help this baby, I implored.

Has he had any mouth sores with the fevers? she asked, seemingly not even hearing what I had said.

What? The question caught me a little off guard, then I realized what she was asking.

No, not that I've noticed, I replied, knowing where she was going with the question this time. See, the *A* in *PFAPA* stands for aphthous stomatitis, or *mouth sores.* According to an article published by the National Center for Biotechnology Information (NCBI) about the prevalence of PFAPA in adults, *Aphthous ulcers, usually on the lips or buccal mucosa, occur in approximately 40-70% of patients* (Ferreira, 2021).

Let's do some math. Since *percent* basically means *out of one hundred*, then 40 to 70% is the equivalent of saying that out of 100 patients (who have been diagnosed with PFAPA) 40 to 70 of them have mouth sores. To break it down even further, if you had a group of ten PFAPA patients in a room and asked them to raise their hand if they ever had mouth sores when their fever spiked, either 4, 5,

6, or (at the most) 7 of them would raise their hands. If you trust that statistic (and it comes from peer-reviewed research so there's not a good reason not to), you have to consider that those other patients who did not raise their hand in our hypothetical survey did *not* have mouth sores. So, out of 10 individuals with PFAPA, at least three (but up to 6) would not have the *A* (aphthous stomatitis), also known as: mouth sores.

That's a pretty significant number of patients that don't have that symptom. As a matter of fact, I would be willing to bet a lot of money (if I was a gambler—oh, and if I had a lot of money) that a person who regularly treated patients with fever disorders came across a few now and again without that symptom. It's just playing the odds.

If Dr. ******* had asked me that question and moved on, I probably wouldn't still be rambling on about the fact that only a percentage of those with PFAPA have that particular symptom which she kept inquiring about. But she didn't move on. She disregarded the fever diary that I had completed with the meticulousness of a surgeon. She ignored the crazy spike in C-reactive protein from the blood draw that she had ordered us to have done when he was in the middle of a fever episode. She showed indifference to my pleas for help, and when I shared with her the research I had read and how Myles' symptoms directly aligned with fever disorders she nodded her head, but said,

When we hear hoof beats, it's usually horses—not zebras. There's a small chance it could be something rare—like a fever disorder—but without the mouth sores it's unlikely. We'll keep watching him. You can bring him back in three months.

Astonishment would probably come closest to describing how I felt in that moment. Of course, the thought that she might not give us a definitive diagnosis had crossed my mind. It was one of my greatest fears about that day—something I had literally had nightmares about in the preceding weeks. But in all honesty, I didn't really *believe* she wouldn't diagnose him. The symptoms lined up. The bloodwork added more proof. The consistency of his episodes sealed it. He had a fever disorder. Why was this *doctor* refusing to help him?

People who know me would probably say I am an introvert. Most often, I would rather listen than talk. (Well, Shawn may not say that, but other people would.) If I had to make a choice between standing up to someone I disagreed with or having my fingernails extracted, it would be a close call. However, there have been a few occasions through the course of my lifetime where I overcame my fear of confrontation, and they all had one thing in common: my kids. If I feel like my kids are being slighted, it makes me upset. This lady was letting my baby boy go for months untreated when she could at least *try* to help him.

Anger kept my nerves at bay as I politely, but firmly, told the doctor that she needed to try treating my son for a fever disorder. I ticked off all of his symptoms again (each of which directly aligned with fever disorders) and I respectfully explained that through the pages of research I had read I knew there was a way to confirm whether or not he had a fever disorder: steroids.

Sounds a little strange, huh? But steroids really could be the answer to our prayers. You see, prednisone (a steroid that is useful in treating inflammation) can be given to a patient who is suspected of having a fever disorder. If the patient does have a fever disorder, the prednisone will bring their fever down in an hour or two. Sometimes, their fever returns the next day. A second dose will almost always take care of it. Fever episode over. Diagnosis confirmed. (Vanoni et al., 2016)

Pleading with Dr. ******* finally prevailed.

We can try *a dose of steroids the next time he has an episode. I suspect it won't work...*

Okay! Yes! I enthusiastically replied. *That's all I want—a chance. If it doesn't work, we can move on.*

I knew it was going to work.

The office visit had felt like what I imagine skydiving would be: terrifying and a little crazy, but with breathtaking exhilaration at the end. Myles had been sick for most of his life and even the doctors didn't know what to do to help him. In my desperation, I had found a possible answer and had somehow talked this doctor into letting us try it. Although we didn't walk out of there with a prescription (or any encouragement that he might get better), we had the promise that we could *try* the medication. Once it worked, we would have a treatment plan. I was flying...but also holding my breath.

GOOD NEWS!

We didn't have to wait long for the opportunity to test my theory. Just like clockwork, Myles started feeling bad. He went to bed. His fever spiked.

This episode (like so many others) began on the weekend. If you are a parent, you know kids are more likely to get sick in the middle of the night or on a Saturday or Sunday. That's just the way it goes. We needed to get the prescription for prednisone, but his regular doctor (the one who suggested that he could have PFAPA) didn't work on weekends. We would have to take him to urgent care and hope for the best. Urgent care is similar to the emergency room. There are great doctors who work there, but there are also *the other kind*. In the words of Forrest Gump, *you never know what you're gonna get*. This is the same facility where I encountered a doctor who told me there was no COVID in our town. No worries, though. We just needed to tell whatever doctor who saw Myles what was going on. All we needed was a couple of doses of prednisone, per Myles' specialist at the University of Kentucky. No problem.

How's it going today? Not feeling too good? the doctor asked as she walked through the door.

No, he feels pretty rough. His temperature went up around three o'clock this morning, I answered her as I held Myles. He was lifeless in my arms, his eyes rolled back. My response didn't really do him justice, but how do you explain how a baby with a 104° fever feels?

How long has it been since he had Tylenol? We need to get some down him...he's pretty hot right now.

Yeah, he was pretty hot. By now I was getting used to the nurses and doctors (who had seen a lot in their years of working with sick people) being shocked by just how hot Myles could get.

We gave him an acetaminophen suppository a couple of hours ago. I told her the same thing I told the nurse.

Let's try some Motrin, then, said the doctor.

I explained that he would throw up the Motrin.

When he's very hot he can't take liquid medication. It also doesn't usually help with his temperature.

Well, let's just try. Sometimes they do better when someone else gives it to them. We've got all kinds of tricks to get the medicine down! The doctor had a smile on her face, and I knew she was trying to be encouraging--friendly even. But I also knew this would just make him more miserable. Regretfully, I did not completely refuse to let them give him the Motrin. Back then, I was still somewhat intimidated by the people who were supposed to be helping my son. Also, I didn't want to seem like a crazy person. I needed her to listen to me. Myles needed prednisone, and since Dr. ******* agreed that we could try it—but didn't give him a prescription—I would have to explain the situation to this doctor and convince *her* to write the prescription.

The affable young nurse walked in carrying a plastic dropperful of the sweet-smelling medicine that the doctor was convinced would cool Myles to a reasonable temperature. Unlike the doctors, the nurses at this office stayed the same. This one was quick with a warm smile. She spoke *to* her young patients, instead of speaking *about* them. While I didn't want anyone bothering Itty, I knew she wanted to help him as she patiently gave him the Motrin drop by drop. And who knows, maybe he'd at least keep it down this—

Bleeeccch...

Every drop that sweet nurse had gotten Myles to swallow came right back up. It barely missed her as she quickly jumped back. It did not miss me or Myles or the floor.

This is when the doctor decided to make her return. She had wanted to get the medicine down so he would start cooling off (104° was not his hottest, but hot enough to be dangerous) so she hadn't examined him or even asked questions yet. The nurse was handing me paper towels as I tried to get the worst off of Itty and I.

You weren't kidding, were you? she quipped as she took in the pink, sticky vomit we were now wearing.

No. He can't take medicine by mouth when he's this hot. The guilt I knew I would feel when I didn't refuse the Motrin was already setting in. Eventually I would learn to say *No!* when it meant protecting him from unnecessary medical procedures, but it's a fine line to refuse treatment when you need them to help your child.

So when did his fever start going up? Now the doctor was ready to talk.

Well, actually, this is normal for him.... I began, explaining his condition to the doctor I had just met just minutes before. I told her about the frequent, consistent fevers, the predictable symptoms: swollen lymph nodes, sore throat, vomiting when the fever first spiked.

We are pretty sure he has a fever disorder. He's seeing a specialist at the University of Kentucky. I was talking fast—part nerves and part fear I wouldn't get it all out before she cut me off. *If it* is *a fever disorder, prednisone will make his fever stop within hours. His doctor said we could try the prednisone, so we just need a prescription for that.* I took a breath. My hands were shaking so I clutched them together as my arms held Myles close.

Well. Let's check him out and then we'll go from there, was the doctor's response.

Her words made me nervous. She didn't immediately agree to give him what he needed, but maybe after she found there was nothing else wrong with him she would understand. It was rare to find a doctor who knew much (if anything at all) about fever disorders, but surely if she didn't believe me, she could call Dr. *******?

Let's get flu, strep, and COVID swabs, she said to the nurse as she began feeling Myles' huge lymph nodes and looking into his throat. The unnecessary tests frustrated me, but we had to prove to her that he didn't have any of the things that came through a doctor's office all day long. Hopefully, this would be the last time I had to put him through this.

Has he been pulling at his ears?

No. Not at all, I informed her.

Okay, she said, *let's wait for the tests to come back and we'll figure out what to do from there*. And she walked out.

Figure out what to do? We *know* what to do. If this doctor wouldn't prescribe his medication we might not be able to get it until his next episode. When Myles is sick, every hour is agonizing. Why won't anybody help?

I can still see the smile on the doctor's face as she walked back into the room. The rest of her fades away, but the smile remains etched in my memory.

Good news! she exclaims.

My heart speeds up. Were we finally, after months and months of trying, going to get him some help?

*I just got off the phone with Dr. ********. Her voice, tinged with an overly cheerful lilt said, *Myles' tests all came back negative, but his ears were pink so we don't need the prednisone—he needs an antibiotic.*

What? My own voice was incredulous, but quiet. In fact, I'm not even sure I spoke the word aloud. I could not believe it. First, that she said he had an ear infection. Second, that she had talked to Dr. *******, the same doctor who had just told me that she would allow us to try a dose of prednisone, and that Dr. ******* had said *not* to try prednisone. And third, that she had prefaced her refusal to help my sick baby with *Good news!* Anger does not come close to explaining how I felt at that moment, but I couldn't find a more appropriate word in the dictionary *or* in the thesaurus, so I'll just use that. I felt extreme anger at the doctor who used his *pink ears* (but were they, really?) as an excuse for his 104° fever. Anger at the *specialist* who not only lied to me, but was for some unknown reason refusing to treat my son. And last, I felt angry with myself. Why was I not able to get Myles the help he needed?

We left the office with a prescription for amoxicillin that I wouldn't fill and instructions to *come back if he doesn't get better.* No, thank you.

SURPRISE TRIP

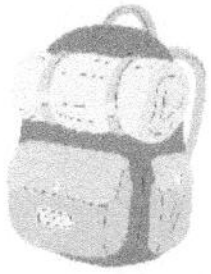

A couple of days later, we were sitting in another room at another medical office. This time (it was a weekday) we were able to get an appointment with Myles' regular pediatrician—the one who had figured out that Myles has a fever disorder and had referred him to the UK Infectious Disease department.

Myles was still running a fever, but he managed a smile as a familiar nurse talked to him and checked his vitals. We had spent a lot of time in this office. My boys liked to guess which animal painting would be on the wall in the room we were led to: baby goats, hens and chicks, or cows. It was usually the cows.

Dr. Avery always knocked before walking in, and this time she had a concerned look on her face. She knew we had been seeing the specialist over the past few months. I believe, like me, she expected to have a resolution to Myles' problem by now. Instead, here we were again, with the same symptoms and no closer to getting him the help he desperately needed.

*Myyy*les...*what are you doing back here?* she sing-songed his name and directed her question to him, though

I would be answering. If a doctor acts like their patient is not in the room (*especially* if said patient is not able to respond), he or she is not a very good doctor.

I explained the past two trips to UK, the research I had done which fully supported the diagnosis she had suggested (PFAPA), and how reluctant Dr. ******* was to treat Myles.

She listened.

With red-rimmed eyes (lack of sleep mixed with being at my emotional breaking point), I relayed my discussion with Dr. ******* about using prednisone to confirm PFAPA—how she had agreed to try it with his next fever—then (after conferring with the doctor at urgent care) refused to let him have it. Myles' pediatrician seemed to be as shocked as I was.

I just don't understand why she won't help him, I complained. *It doesn't make any sense. I'm not asking her to do some million-dollar testing on him, or give him a controlled substance. Why is she so against trying to treat my baby?* It was out of character for me to be so vocal about my lack of faith in one medical practitioner to *another* medical practitioner (the one who sent me to her, as a matter of fact), but this whole experience had changed me.

Myles needed me to stand up for him, so I was going to push until someone helped him.

I don't understand either, Myles' doctor replied honestly.

Those few words made me feel less crazy. They validated my feelings about the disregard Dr. ******* had shown my son. I wasn't the only one who saw it.

We were both quiet as she began examining Myles. He was so hot. He didn't protest as I gently jostled him around to let her look at one ear, then the other.

Tell me again, what was their reasoning for denying the prednisone? she asked.

The urgent care doctor said he had an ear infection. She prescribed antibiotics. But, honestly, I didn't fill them... My voice trailed off as I expected to be reprimanded for ignoring the doctor's orders.

I continued, *When the urgent care doctor looked at his ears, she didn't say anything about them looking infected, so I was shocked when she came back in the room and said they were pink. He hadn't been pulling at them or acting like they hurt, at all.* I justified my actions (not giving him the antibiotics) because I cared what this person—the one doctor who had really tried to help Myles—thought about me. *That doctor just said he had an ear infection after* *she had called Dr.* *******. *It was like they were looking for an excuse to tell me we couldn't try the steroids. Have his ears gotten worse? I know I should've given him the antibiotics but I really thought they were just...*

I only stopped rambling when the pediatrician interrupted me, *His ears look perfect.*

Perfect? I questioned. *Perfect?* Was I hearing her correctly?

Yes, she reaffirmed. *They look great.*

A flood of emotions overtook me as I realized what she was telling me. We seem to naturally put such faith in these professionals--these men and women who are so much smarter than we are, who go to school for years and years before they assume their position. Our lives (and the lives of our children and all those we love) are placed in their capable hands. You hear stories about nurses who murder newborn babies and doctors who inject air into the IV's of the elderly, but it doesn't truly shake your belief in medical professions until it happens to you. Or to someone you love. Those *stories* are like fairy tales. You know they happened, but they would never happen to *you.* Granted, my baby was alive (which I thank God for every day), but the extreme temperatures that he endured monthly (at minimum) could have taken his life or caused irreversible damage to his brain. God was taking care of Myles. The doctors were gambling with his life every time they sent us home without treatment.

Once I regained my ability to speak, the questions rushed out, *Why would she do this? Why won't she diagnose him? Or even let him try prednisone? If we're wrong about it being PFAPA, then we can move on. Try something else. But she won't try anything! Why is she doing this to us?*

I don't know. I really thought he would be diagnosed by now, the pediatrician's honest reply, again, was grounding. It was a breath of fresh air. I was at my breaking point. I worried about Myles all the time. He would be sick for days, we would get a few days (at the most three weeks) to recover, then he was sick again. We slept when he was well. We survived when he wasn't. Now, while holding my very sick little boy, I have just learned that Dr. ******* never really intended to let us try the medication that could help him, and that another doctor has seemingly conspired with her to create an *ear infection* as an excuse to break her word.

From the outside looking in, it would be so easy to say *why didn't you file a complaint? Get a lawyer! File a lawsuit!* Me from the present can judge what I did back then with ease. I probably should have done a lot of things differently. But when you're going through it....

I have an idea... Dr. Avery began, *maybe Dr.* ******* *just needs to see him when he's like this. He's never been to an appointment with her when he was actively in an episode, has he?*

No, I responded, wondering where she was going with this. Maybe she was going to try to get him an appointment coinciding with a future episode? I started to reach for my phone so I could pull up my calendar...but did I even want to go back to Dr. ******* again? I quickly made a decision to give her one more chance. Maybe Dr. Avery was right and she needed to see how sick Myles got with an episode.

Would you be opposed to taking him to UK hospital, having him admitted, if we can work it out?

Yes! I mean—no--I wouldn't be opposed... You mean...today? I questioned.

My sleep-deprived brain was trying to jump ahead to figuring out the logistics as I listened to her. What about the boys? Shawn and I wouldn't leave them anywhere, but that would mean I'd have to go alone, which was not the best situation when he was this sick. But of course I'd have to go alone—the pandemic. Only one parent would be allowed in. How long would they keep him? What if Dr. ******* refused to accept him?

Dr. Avery was crafting the plan as she talked. Her determination to get help for my son was evident as she devised how to get Dr. ******* to see what was really going on with him.

My heart pounded as she left the room to try to make arrangements for Myles to be admitted into the UK hospital. Quickly and quietly, I took out my phone and called Shawn.

I think Dr. Avery is sending us to UK. Today.

Today? he questioned. *What's happened?* Shawn's voice was suddenly bordering on frantic. Myles had been so sick so many times, but we were usually sent home after our appointment.

Nothing's changed, I told him. *She thinks if Dr. ******* sees him during an episode, she will have to realize what it is and do something. That she'll actually diagnose him so he can get treatment.*

That's great! They have to help him, baby. This is so hard on him.

Oh! And, his ears were fine. They weren't infected. As I repeated it to my husband, I felt both shock and validation.

What do you mean, his ears are fine? His voice was questioning, but not angry. Yet.

Dr. Avery looked in both ears. Then she looked again. She said "his ears are perfect."

But they said he had an ear infection? That's why they wouldn't give him the medicine.

It was like I could hear the gears moving as the realization came to him. *So that doctor lied to you? Is that what happened? She just didn't want him to have the prednisone or what?* Now. Now his voice was angry.

I didn't even fill the antibiotics. They don't get better that quickly. Especially with no antibiotics, I said to myself as well as Shawn.

We were silent for a moment. That was probably better than saying the things we were thinking about the doctor who claimed he had ear infections (*Good news!*) and the specialist who refused to treat him.

I broke the silence when I remembered what I needed to ask, *Can you pack for us? If this works out I'll need to hurry. I want to get there before dark. I can run by the house—get our bags and kiss the boys—then we'll be on the way.*

Wait a minute—he started then stopped. *I mean, yeah, of course I'll get everything ready. But you can't take the baby by yourself. What if something happens while you're on the interstate? You can't drive and watch him at the same time.*

He was too worried to tease me about what we were both actually thinking—I am (as my son, Caleb, once put it so eloquently) *geographically challenged*. I once got lost in our small town going to pick up an order at the local restaurant.

They won't let us both in. And you have to watch the boys. We can't leave them overnight.

I'll drive you.

But, Shawn. They won't let us both stay. And I'm not leaving Myles.

I'll drive you, he repeated. *Call your sister. Ask her to watch the boys. I'll take you and Myles then I'll come home after I know you all are safe and sound.*

As we waited, I rocked Myles and I prayed. The rocking was as much for me as it was him. The prayers were for my family, for God to work everything out, and for Shawn and I to be able to do what we needed to do. And with every quick breath Myles breathed, I prayed a silent thank you to God.

Dr. Avery had it all worked out. Myles would go to the emergency department at UK hospital, and they would admit him when a bed became available. Myles' episodes usually lasted an average of four to five days (though he's had some that lasted a whole week—and occasionally one would be as short as two days), so he should be headed towards the end of this one. Normally, that would be a good thing, but we needed Dr. ******* to see him at his worst. This felt like our last chance. Every few weeks (or days) we went from sailing on calm waters to being tossed about by thrashing waves, barely able to stay above the surface. I wanted Dr. ******* to reach out her hand and pull us up. Would she do it? Or would she just let us keep struggling for air?

Hailey lived on campus at UK. She had decided to meet us at the hospital to see Myles before we went in. Surprisingly, the hospital staff allowed her to accompany us into the emergency department.

How's he doing? Hailey asked as we followed the nurse to an ER exam room.

He slept until we got about twenty minutes out. Then he threw up. Car rides are hard on him.

Yeah, you and me both, dude, she addressed Myles.

*His fever's down some today. I just hope and pray Dr. ******* will do something.*

She's got to.... Hailey had been looking into fever disorders, too. She didn't get to be with Myles as much as she would like, but as a student in the health field she had access to more research journals than I did, so she had done her share of investigating. Hailey had come to the same conclusion that I had: Myles had PFAPA, and he needed prednisone to confirm it.

Spending the night in a hospital is about as much fun as going to the gynecologist. If you're there, you are either sick, or you're with someone you really love who is sick. Or you're pregnant. So unless you are there to give birth, you would probably rather be literally anywhere else in the world. But honestly, as much as I didn't want to be there, part of me felt like a kid on Christmas Eve (would we finally get the gift we've been waiting for...a diagnosis?). The other part of me felt like I was walking toward the gallows. My body was like a live wire, my neck stiff with tension, and my nerves raw. Tremors made my hands betray how I was surviving on caffeine, sleeping for minutes at a time while Myles was laying on my chest.

So many times I had anticipated a resolution. This time, in fleeting moments I let myself believe, in between much longer moments of fearing being sent away yet again. We had been hopeful and then been let down over and over. Every time I took him to a doctor, I had some expectation that they would help him. Was my faith strong enough to do it one more time?

Shawn had said once, *For a woman who has so much faith in God, you worry a lot. You need to trust Him. He's always taken care of us and He always will.* I was stunned. Speechless. He was absolutely right. God had *always* taken care of us. He has plans for us that we would never imagine. It is so very easy to trust Him when everything is sunshine and rainbows. Not so easy when it's darkness and pain. But He always has us in His hands. He always has a plan.

He's always taken care of us and He always will.

HAVE YOU EVER HEARD OF PFAPA?

Why, yes. Yes, I have.

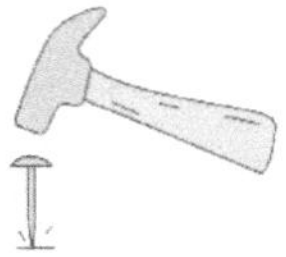

One of the residents that had come in to check on Myles had asked me a question, but I must have misheard her. I really needed to get a little sleep.

I'm sorry? What did you ask me? In addition to my mind exhibiting the lethargy my body felt, the masks we were wearing made communication more difficult.

I asked if you've ever heard of PFAPA? It's a fever disorder? From looking at his history and his chart, he must have one.

Hailey sat up from her reclined position, leaning forward to join the conversation.

That's...actually why they're here. Hailey glanced at me with a hopeful look. The doctor could've just told us we might have the winning lottery numbers. I was suddenly wide awake from the surge of adrenaline.

He has all the hallmark symptoms of PFAPA—that's the most common fever disorder in his demographic. The resident stated this as commonly known information, just like she would've said, *It's really been a nice day out there, hasn't it?*

Taking in my confused look, she asked, *Has he not been diagnosed with it yet?*

No...but that's what we think he has. His pediatrician thinks it's what he's got. He's just sick so often. And his fevers are like, on schedule. Like, we know when his next one will be. They're always the same. He has the same symptoms every time. Like every three weeks. My ability to communicate coherently was somewhat diminished by the shock of what she was saying.

When she left the room, Hailey and I just stared at each other.

I asked, *Did she really just say he has PFAPA?*

I mean, basically, yeah. She said he has all the symptoms.

She literally just met him. She looked at his chart and talked to us for what—two minutes?—and she figured out that he has it. Why is it taking his SPECIALIST months to admit that's what he has? My elation at the resident's declaration was mixed with anger at his doctor for not seeing what was right in front of her. I was beginning to think maybe she did see it. Was there another reason she was refusing to diagnose him?

The following hours were some of the worst of my life. Even with the proof right in front of her, Dr. ******* had a battery of tests ordered for Itty to undergo. Reliving that part of Myles' journey makes my stomach hurt. Especially now, a couple of years later, I believe putting him through those tests was cruel. Maybe even sadistic. Someone is probably experiencing the same thing right now, which is disgusting. Unnecessary tests. Worse because it happens to babies, to children. Add in that they are already sick and feeling at their worst and it is just heartbreaking.

When I was at Vanderbilt in preterm labor (over twenty years ago), they did a urine catheter to see if I had a kidney infection. After, I told someone that I would rather go through childbirth than have that done again. At that time, I had never been through childbirth so it was an easy statement for me to make. Now I've done it five times. I only had an epidural once (it was too late—I was pushing by the time they finished), and the others went too fast to even try to get one. Today, I stand by my original statement. At least after childbirth you end up with a baby. The other experience is painful, humiliating, and has little to no benefit. They did that to my baby. They held him down and did a urine cath. The nurse asked if I wanted to leave the room, but I stayed. I looked into his eyes and held his tiny hand. I had allowed them to put him through this, so I didn't break eye contact as he screamed, *mommmyyy.* I allowed *all* those tests she ordered because for some reason she wanted to do those tests before she would diagnose him. Even though he had had 103° to 105° temperatures on a regular schedule since he was three months old. Even though we knew what he had, his pediatrician knew what he had, and a resident who glanced at his chart knew what he had. We all knew he didn't have a kidney infection. We knew what the bloodwork would show because he had had more blood draws in his short life than I had in my 40-something years. But I let her do it. He suffered through those tests because I, his mother, allowed it. I let her have her fun this one last time so she would finally admit that he had a fever disorder. Because then, and only then, could we get him some relief.

After a few hours, a nurse came in to tell me they had a room available and would be moving us out of the emergency department. Since he was being officially admitted, Hailey's welcome was rescinded and she was escorted out as we were escorted up (in a wheelchair, of course). Funny, they had no worries about putting Myles through tests that could have actual risks, but once he was admitted the biggest concern was that I would fall and injure him while carrying him up to the room. Not that I minded the ride by that point in the evening.

Once we were upstairs, a whole new set of doctors, nurses, CNA's, RNA's, residents, interns, PA's, and XYZ's paraded through to meet us and explain who they were and what they did. I *wish* I was exaggerating, but, you know: teaching hospital. The introvert in me was so far past the end of my rope that the last unraveling thread was cutting into my fingers as I tried to hold on. The muscles in my face hurt from plastering on a smile for each new person I had to meet, as I answered the same questions over and over in hopes that *this* would be the one who would help Myles. The resident's words from hours earlier sustained me. If *she* saw it, then maybe they would, too.

A hospital never sleeps, but the procession finally ended, and for a few hours in the dead of night we were only visited by a couple of nurses making their hourly rounds. One of those sweet ladies had brought me an extra pillow. I propped it under my left arm, raised the metal guardrail on that side, and snuggled Myles against me. I breathed him in as the rise and fall of his chest lulled me to sleep.

THE LAST DANCE

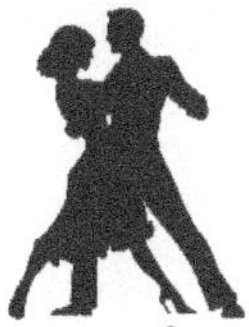

My babies have always had the ability to knock me out faster than a shot of NyQuil. If you've ever breastfed a baby, then you know what I'm talking about. And while I know the technical reason that I can't keep my eyes open when I'm nursing (the act of breastfeeding causes the hormones prolactin and oxytocin—the *love* hormone—to be released, which makes the nursing mama relaxed and sleepy), I believe it's more than the science behind it. You have that warm little baby laying on you, feeling his tiny, rhythmic heartbeat as you inhale that sweet scent that can only be described as *baby...* it just does something to you. If you've never breastfed, I would compare it to laying on your favorite beach, the breeze cooling your skin as you listen to the waves lapping against the shore. Not to say I've done that. Anytime I've been at the beach I was chasing kids. But I imagine it's something like that.

I can't sleep through the night without checking a few times to make sure my kids are breathing. *Especially* when they're babies. So being able to feel Myles' breath rise and fall against me was really the only way I could fully relax enough to sleep.

But, you know, we *were* in a hospital. So even though I went to sleep pretty quickly, I woke up even quicker. I might've slept an hour if you took all the minutes and put them together. Itty, however, slept better than he had since his fever spiked a few days before.

And now, his fever was gone.

Even though the purpose of bringing Myles to UK was so Dr. ******* could see him during the height of an episode, she had not seen him during the height (nor any other part) of the episode. No big deal, though. It's not like we rushed to a town two hours away, with a sick baby who vomited because he gets carsick—even on short trips—to see a doctor who lives minutes from the hospital, who couldn't be bothered to come to the hospital in the first 12 hours he was there when he actually *did* still have a fever. Oh, wait, it was actually exactly like that.

Now, I know I sound a little resentful, or *salty,* as my kids would say (they're probably already onto a new word by now, but you get it), so I feel like I need to add qualifiers here. Doctors are such important members of society. They save lives. I sincerely appreciate what they do. *Grey's Anatomy* was one of my favorite shows (until they killed off Derek—unnecessary and, in my opinion, ruined the show). Medical professionals save people's lives every single day.

They put their own health and families on the back burner to help others. I just want to make it clear that I truly, wholeheartedly respect those who serve in the medical field. They do things for strangers that most people wouldn't want to do for their best friends. And I haven't even mentioned the emotional investment that many of these special people put into what they do. Especially the nurses. Let's be honest, nurses usually do the lion's share of the hands-on work. They celebrate with you when there's good news, and comfort you in mourning and through pain. For every bad apple in the medical profession, there's a thousand good ones.

So our *apple* showed up late that afternoon, after Myles had entertained the nurses with his songs and conversation and was feeling like a million dollars.

She had an entourage of medical students and residents with her. I had Itty wiggling restlessly in my arms. My heartbeat sped up, and I got palpitations like I used to when my ex-husband would decide to come around to visit the kids. Back then I used anti-anxiety meds to try to control my nerves. Now I did breathing exercises and held Myles close. Usually that worked. This time, it didn't.

Well, he looks like he feels better. Her words were friendly, but her expression was foreboding. It said *I would rather be anywhere else than in this room, talking to this woman.*

Ironically, I suddenly felt the same way.

Yeah, he, um...his fever broke last night. This one lasted about four days. Now he'll feel great until, well...about three weeks from now. That's the current pattern. I was hoping you could see him when he was hot but I—

I'm glad he's feeling better. She cut me off mid-sentence. To be fair, I guess I *was* rambling a little bit.

This is my resident, Dr. Sebastian. He'll be going over your son's test results.

The young man in the khakis and white lab coat made eye contact with me.

Hello, I'm Dr. Sebastian. Nice to meet you, he politely raised his hand to offer a fist bump—the official handshake of the 2020's.

His eyes were kind and his voice was steady. Look closer, though, and you could see that he hadn't been a doctor long enough to be completely sure of himself. He had a supervisor, and she was in the room watching him. As a new teacher back then, I could sympathize with him. Even if you *know* you're doing everything like you should, it is harrowing to have a superior watching and critiquing you like Ebert used to critique movies.

So Dr. ******* had put this young doctor up to *review your son's* (Myles. His name is Myles. It's right there on the chart.) *test results.* The way she had said it gave me pause. She knew I wanted to know the name of the condition that was causing his fevers. Instead, she was having someone else *go over test results.* Was she so opposed to admitting that she was wrong that she was having her subordinate talk for her? She couldn't even say *your son has a fever disorder*?

He continued, *As you know, we did a lot of tests...blood labs, urine* (Oh yes, I know. I will never forget.), *flu, strep, COVID...and a complete respiratory panel.*

I sat quietly while he talked. Myles had latched onto me to nurse, so he was still, too. My heart was doing somersaults but my body wasn't moving. (That's not entirely true. My hands trembled, but they clutched Itty so no one could see.)

So we did all of this because of your concerns...he has *been sick pretty frequently...and his fever was reported to be fairly high* (Reported? His fever was almost 105°. Monica, do *not* respond. Wait until he's finished. You'll sound like a crazy person.) *So, we did find something.*

This is the moment we've been waiting for. We've been doing this for about a year and a half, but it feels like we've been waiting a lifetime for a resolution. For about thirty percent of Myles' life (if you take the bad days and combine them) he's been so sick he couldn't hold his head up. So when he said *we did find something* I got one of those physical shocks—I don't know how to explain it, but if you've had it, you know. I got the same feeling the first time Shawn looked into my eyes and said my name. The feeling is seared into my brain but I don't have the words to describe it. Some people call it *butterflies*, but a thousand butterflies couldn't make me feel the way this did.

Now I think he was waiting for me to ask, *What did you find*, but I couldn't speak. Time stopped. Those somersaults my heart was doing must have been contagious because they went to my brain. It was thinking so many things at once: *They're finally going to help him...I can't wait to tell Shawn...and Melinda...and mom...I should call Hailey...Now I need to research treatments... Caleb and Cash and Max will be thrilled... Will they give him medicine today, or wait until the next episode...*

Seconds later, he continued. I felt awkward making direct eye contact with this doctor, but I wanted to let him know I was focused on what he was saying.

So I don't know if you know what a respiratory panel is? But it tests for around twenty viruses and bacterial infections. It's the test they did when they put the q-tip up his nose? We did that because it gives us a lot of answers and shows things we can't really identify with certainty any other way...

I nodded my head, not because I understood why he was talking about a respiratory panel or how that panel could identify PFAPA, but so he would keep going.

Well. The panel showed that Myles (the resident had at least learned my *son's* name) *has rhinovirus.*

Again, I nodded so he would continue. He didn't.

Finally, I responded, *Okay, so he has rhinovirus. That's a common cold, right?*

That is the virus that causes the common cold. Right. A female resident had answered me while the room stayed silent.

Well, we know that wouldn't cause his high fevers. And it's not like you can get a common cold on a regular schedule and then turn it off and feel great. So: did you find out what is *causing his fevers that are occurring on a REGULAR SCHEDULE?* My voice was a little shaky, but had started off quiet and composed. As I spoke, however, it increased in both volume and pitch. Surely, they had much more to tell me—*like a diagnosis*—and he had just paused for dramatic effect?

In some cases, rhinovirus can lead to other illnesses—like pneumonia—and that can *cause high fevers.* This time, the ringleader herself spoke. Her voice betrayed no emotion. Her eyes were cold.

But he doesn't have pneumonia, now, does he? This makes no sense. I know you aren't trying to tell me that the months and months of fevers—THAT I CAN PREDICT CORRECTLY ON A CALENDAR—are because he tested positive for a common cold during this one. What were his SED rates? What about his CRP?

Again, silence. After what felt like forever, someone finally spoke.

Let me see... We were back to the young resident to whom Dr. ******* had given the reins. He was quickly tapping on his black iPad, which until now had been hiding at his side under some papers. *Okay, here it is...*

He gave me the C-reactive protein result first. Myles' CRP was *ridiculously* high. The doctor didn't say that, though. He didn't give me a reference range. He just gave me the number and said, *it's a little elevated.* CRP was such a big part of many of the journal articles I read on fever disorders. I was very familiar with the range which would be considered normal. Myles' CRP was nowhere near that range. His score had run past the top range, taken an Uber to the airport, flown halfway around the world, then hopped onto a space shuttle.

And his SED rate? I prompted him.

Although the doctor's name (*Sebastian*) had Greek origins, I believe he had a little Irish in him. Red crept up his neck and to his ears as he read off the result. It felt like deja vu' (but just from a few seconds ago) as he told me the SED rate was *a little elevated.*

As I've said before, I am not a confrontational person. But throw my kids into the mix and all bets are off. I was so tired of this woman standing between my son and his treatment.

I took a long, deep breath as the fifteen hundred doctors in the room looked at me as though my skin had turned blue and I had sprouted wings. The female resident who had responded to my question about rhinovirus (really it was more of a statement—I knew it was a common cold—but at least she was brave enough to acknowledge that's what it was) made eye contact with me and I could feel the connection. She knew I was being bamboozled. It didn't take a rocket scientist (or a doctor with decades of medical school and experience) to see that all the facts were laid out in front of us, but were (for some unknown reason) being ignored. My one-year-old little boy was taking the hit for whatever this doctor's crazy problem was.

Okay. So his SED rate and CRP are elevated. He has fevers that occur regularly—with the same symptoms every time: high fever, swollen lymph nodes, sore throat, and vomiting. The fevers last three to five days, then he makes a full recovery. I can actually write down on the calendar when his next fever will be—within a day or two—and that is when he gets a fever. But you want me to believe that a COLD is causing this particular fever. AND WHAT MADE HIM SICK THE OTHER FORTY TIMES HE HAD A FEVER SO HIGH HE COULD GET BRAIN DAMAGE?

I wasn't yelling, but my voice had risen enough that I would not be surprised if they had triggered something to summon a security guard. Itty Bear tightened his grip on me. His eyes had closed when he latched on, and he squeezed them tightly shut. It was one of his coping mechanisms when he wanted to escape the doctors—he would hide in my shirt or under a blanket and shut the world out.

None of the underlings would look at me. For a few seconds, you could've heard a pin drop. But Dr. ******* wasn't going to back down. She had made her decision and *who was I* to talk back to *her*, a doctor—a specialist even—with years of experience.

Look, I know you would like for me to say your son has some rare disorder. But it's just like I told you before: when you hear hoof beats it's usually a horse, not a zebra. Children get viruses, and your son...(at this point I wanted to lay Myles, M-Y-L-E-S, *Myles* on the bed, pick up the closest, heavy object I could grab—any metal bedpans lying around?—and launch it directly at that woman's head) *....apparently gets a lot of viruses.*

She could have been saying the pledge to the Russian flag in Dutch after that and I would not have heard a word of what she had said. Her voice had turned to white noise—you know, the sound we used to hear when the cable went out (if you're under 40, ask a grown up what I'm talking about).

After she decided to double down on her misinformed, preposterous "diagnosis," I was no longer interested in anything she had to say. I had given this lady chance after chance after chance, and I was done. Her actions (or lack thereof) had made me literally consider violence (like, to the point of thinking about the logistics and repercussions before completely ruling it out). I needed to get out of that situation as quickly as possible.

This was not me. I was neither violent nor inclined to have a temper. But I felt like I was beating my head against a brick wall and nothing was happening. (What does that saying mean, anyway? Why would someone beat their head against *anything*—much less a brick wall—and expect something good to happen?) I could scream and beg and cry for help from this doctor for my son—my *baby*—but it would not make any difference. She was not going to help him.

This was not the way the world was supposed to work. Though life had taught me some very cold lessons about trusting *anyone* (there is only one you can ever fully trust, and that is God), I still had the belief that those who had answered the call to be doctors and nurses and *community helpers* (that's the kindergarten teacher coming out) were basically good people. They would help those in need, right? At every turn, Dr. ******* had chipped away at my trust in the medical system. She had made me almost lose one of the most important things you can ever have: faith.

Now, I know that Dr. ******* was not the only person to let us down on this journey. There were doctors who diagnosed Myles with things he didn't have. There were nurses who treated me like a liar when I told them what his temperature had been, and how often he had been sick. There were people who acted like I was crazy or making up symptoms (some professionals, others not). But Dr. ******* was the one who truly made me *feel* crazy. She was supposed to be this highly acclaimed professional. She had years of experience and she had students or recent graduates working under her at each meeting we had. All her accolades and experience and subordinates made me feel inferior. By the way she talked to me, it also made her feel superior.

Until that very last visit, I was convinced that she knew more about my son's medical condition than I did, but more importantly than that, I believed that she would try to help him. Yes, I got angry with her at the earlier visits. Even through my anger, I thought she was just going through the process, and that her intention was to figure out what was causing Myles to be sick. Even though I saw all the signs, she was the professional and saw hundreds of sick children every month. Maybe she just needed more evidence before she was convinced?

Looking back, I think I just could not comprehend that a medical doctor would maliciously fail to diagnose a child, and in doing so allow him to continue to be deathly sick over and over. There is sin in this world and people can do terrible things to each other. The thing is, it's more comprehensible to the human mind that *people in New York City rob and kill each other* and *if girls go to frat parties they're going to get raped*, than *my child's teacher sent nude photos to her classmate* or *my baby's doctor wanted him to stay sick.* We love watching crime shows about the horrible, shocking things humans do to other people, but we never truly believe it can happen to us. It's all sin. It does happen. When it touches you or someone you love, it changes your whole worldview. It changes *you.*

Once I realized that Dr. ******* was not going to help Myles, I was ready to get out of there. She seemed to be as anxious as I was to part ways. It had taken her almost twenty-four hours to come to Myles' bedside. Her exit, in contrast, was so expeditious it would've been comical if it wasn't so sad.

Such a large group of white coats had converged on us. They all seemed to be as ready as Dr. ******* was to make their escape. The young female doctor who had affirmed my comment about rhinovirus, however, lagged behind.

She made eye contact with me. The salty, angry tears that I had refused to let fall escaped as I glanced away to avoid her stare.

This. Is not. Because. Of a cold. The words escaped through my clenched teeth. I hated how furious my voice sounded. Myles was still in my arms and I knew he could feel the venom radiating from my soul.

She was at least ten years my junior. Her makeup and hair were perfection (I had "slept" in a hospital bed underneath Itty, and my hair hadn't seen a brush or a flat iron in days). If this *person* tried to convince me that a cold could make my baby run a 104.8° fever...

I was past my breaking point. I didn't trust myself. *Dear God, please help me to not do something stupid.*

You know, you're doing the right thing, the young physician began.

I'm not doing anything, I replied. *My son needs help and I am not helping him. I am failing him. Over and over. How can that be the right thing?*

You are fighting for him.

She was on my side? Her compassionate eyes had hinted at that earlier, but when she stayed behind I assumed she just wanted to convince me that her mentor was right—that Myles just caught a lot of viruses and that he did not have some strange disorder that caused fevers on a regular basis.

You are his mother. You know him better than anyone. Her sideways glances toward the open door exposed her apprehension of Dr. ******* returning and overhearing our conversation. She still stayed.

This is not normal, I insisted. *I can predict his next fever every time.* My voice was raspy. Pleading. My hands still shook, but I felt more confident than ever that I had to keep going.

*You know, when we got to the ER yesterday—before he got a room—there was a doctor...she had looked at his chart and the first thing she asked me was if I had heard of fever disorders. She hadn't spent five minutes with him and she knew what it was. I don't understand why Dr. ******* won't admit he has PFAPA. He can't get treated because she wants to pretend this is normal. This is NOT normal.* I inhaled sharply to steady myself, and to give her a chance to speak.

*No, it's not normal. But in my opinion, Dr. ******* has made up her mind, and she is not one to be swayed.*

So what do I do? I am not *giving up.* Of that, I was certain, but where could I go from here? Dr. ******* was a specialist with years and years of both education and experience. She was currently (according to her own words) very influential in Kentucky's fight against COVID

19. Not only that, but she was also an extremely prominent staff member at the University of Kentucky hospital. It's not like I could just change doctors.

You keep going. The doctor's gaze drifted over toward the door again, but her voice was unfaltering. *Take him somewhere else. And if that doesn't work—* she paused. *It'll work. They'll see. But if they don't, then don't stop. You will find an answer. And one day, he'll know you fought for him.*

Some people never know what they've done for you. How they've made your day better, pulled you off the ledge, perhaps even altered the entire trajectory of your life. On that day, October 24th, 2020, a young doctor gave me the determination I needed to keep fighting the system. Her fearlessness gave me courage. Ever so much more importantly, her heart restored my faith. While her image used to be vividly emblazoned in my memory, the years have caused it to fade like a favorite jean jacket. Nevertheless, while we were only together in that room for a few minutes, she made an impression on my life (and on Myles') that will never be forgotten.

LETTING GO

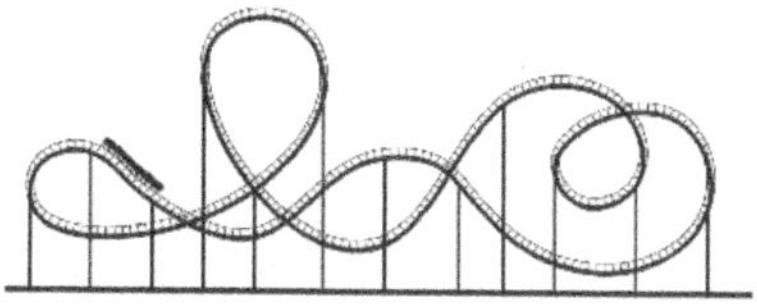

The days following Myles' stint at UK, as I tried to map out our next steps, evoke memories of our ride on the iconic roller coaster at the pier in Santa Monica. Salt water (and a hint of cinnamon) scented the air, and for a few seconds, I felt like I was flying over the Pacific Ocean. Wait a minute... That's not how it reminded me of that roller coaster...

Let me try again. In those days, my emotions ranged from apprehensive to elated, as well as everything in between. I remember being so excited as I anticipated the quick thrill of soaring around the track. Then, as Cash and Max climbed into the coaster seat my anxiety spiked. *What if the bar came loose? What if Cash couldn't hold onto Max* (he was barely at the height limit anyway) *and Max flew out? What if? What if? What if?* When I remembered to put my faith in God, I felt secure, protected, and happy. At peace. Once I let the doubts come in, (*What if he never gets a diagnosis? What if one of these crazy high fevers causes brain damage?*) It was like that gradual, creeping train crawling up the track. With every inch, with every doubt, my fear grew. *Danger was coming*. Then, I would remember that God is in control, and as the coaster train flew down the other side, I released the fear and doubt, and let the peace in.

When Hailey and Caleb were little, they had a videotape (I know, I'm old.) of the VeggieTales. There was a little vegetable (I think he was a toddler zucchini, but he might have been broccoli) who was scared of the dark. The wise tomato and the silly cucumber went to visit him during the night. They had a wonderful conversation and then they all ended up singing a rollicking song together. You know, because that's what you do when two grown men—I mean, vegetables—show up in a little boy's bedroom in the middle of the night. They sang, *God is bigger than the boogie man. He's bigger than Godzilla or the monsters on t.v.* And yes, I sang that as I wrote it and I will probably be singing it all day now.

I have sung that song to all five of my children. Some have heard it as they were being rocked to sleep. Others, when they have been afraid of the dark or worried about a school bully. If you don't have small children, someone may look at you funny if you burst out in song, *God is bigger than the boogie man...* However, the message is clear and true no matter your age: God is bigger than anything. He is bigger than anyone. He can *do* anything. Our nature as humans allows us to worry when something goes wrong, but our place as God's children allows us to trust in Him and know it is all going to be okay. As therapist and Christian and rock climber Lonnie Jones once said, *what can they do to me? Cut my head off? Okay. I'm going home to Jesus!*

As a mom, I am going to worry about my kids. Not being able to get help for Myles was a very difficult time in our lives with a lot of slow scary hills to climb. But every time I remembered to put my faith in God and trust that he was going to lead us on the right path, I felt that sweet release of letting go. Just like flying through the air on an iconic coaster.

CALM AND ACCEPTING

Oh, wait, I meant the opposite.

A cold? What do you mean—she said he had a COLD? My daughter, Hailey, did not get her personality from me. While I would rather chew off my own arm than to argue with someone, Hailey lives for the opportunity. It's really a shame her high school didn't have a debate team.

Hailey was livid. Although she doesn't get to spend a considerable amount of time with Myles, she was there at his birth. Seeing a new life make its way into the world is an incredible thing. A miracle right before your eyes. Hailey will always feel a connection to her youngest baby brother. So when I relayed Dr. *******'s "diagnosis", my eldest (and only) daughter was not happy.

She. Did not. Say that. Hailey challenged.

Yes, Hailey, she did. She had her lackey explain it to me like it was a good *thing. Like, guess what? Something showed up!* my voice teeming with sarcasm.

There was contempt in hers as she shot back, *what is* wrong *with her?*

I don't—

She is supposed to be one of the top doctors in the state! A COLD? Hailey's voice was so loud the kids could hear every word she was saying through the phone. *He had a hundred and five degree fever!*

Well, actually it was only 104.8 this time, so—

Oh! 104.8! Is that all? He could have a febrile seizure, mother. It is extremely dangerous for any*one to have a fever that high! Much less, my one-year-one baby brother. That "doctor" doesn't know what she's talking about.* Hailey's caustic tone conveyed some of the emotions I was feeling as well. Nevertheless, I felt compelled to try and calm her down. After all, she was a student in the heath field at UK and could be negatively affected if Dr. ******* found out she was saying such disparaging things about her. Last thing I wanted was for that woman to hurt *two* of my children.

Look! Right here! She had switched us to FaceTime and was jabbing her finger at her iPad screen.

Cold symptoms: Sneezing. Stuffy nose. Watery eyes. Has he had any of those? Then, (without waiting for me to respond) *Mucus draining from nose and/or throat. Any mucus? No? You know what* isn't *listed here? Ridiculously high fever. Not listed. I believe Dr. ******* needs to go back to medical school before she-*

Hailey. That's enough. I know you're upset. Believe me, I am furious. But getting angry isn't going to help us and it really *isn't going to help Myles. We are going to find someone who will help him. I am not giving up.*

Well, that woman is ridiculous. And she teaches other doctors! Do you know how many up-and-coming medical professionals she influences every day? We have to do something....

I jumped in quickly and interjected, *Actually, she may not have as much influence as you think.*

What do you mean? She has residents under her all the time. Maybe that's *why she got divorced....* Hailey mumbled the last part, but I felt like I had to get her off the topic of Dr. ******* before someone overheard her.

*Hailey! Stop worrying about Dr. ******* and listen for a minute.*

I'm just saying....

Hailey!

Okay, mother. Say what you want to say, The exasperation in her voice was a throwback to a teenager trying to explain new technology to a parent or complaining about their curfew being earlier than their friends'.

I recounted what happened with the resident who stayed behind to encourage me to seek help elsewhere. Hailey, who (I can say this because she's mine and I love her) is not always the best listener, silently took in every word. When I finished, I took a grounding breath and awaited her response.

Well.

This was the equivalent of speechlessness for my daughter.

Yeah....

That's a really big deal. I mean....do you know how residency works?

Um. I know the residents are like, under the attendings. I know she took a big risk talking to me, I answered.

So, all of the residents have graduated from medical school, but they still have to complete a residency before they're on their own. Technically, a resident can't do anything without approval from their attending. So even if allll of those residents in the boy's room believed he had PFAPA, it wouldn't matter because that woman (she said *woman* like it tasted like soured milk) *refuses to admit he has it. And she's in charge.*

Yeah, I get that part...

*Furthermore, if Dr. ******* had heard one of her residents essentially saying she was wrong, it could really make her angry. She could cause that resident a lot of trouble for the rest of her time at UK. And that could be months. Or years. She could even cause the resident to not get a fellowship or a job later on. Think of it like when you were student teaching and you had a supervising teacher.*

Both of mine were great, I interjected.

Yeah, but if one of them hadn't been, and if you made them mad, all your college work and your future career could have gone down the drain. I know a normal person wouldn't do that to someone, but we're talking about a doctor who doesn't want to help a toddler get better. She could do a lot of damage if she had overheard that resident talking to you. Just depends on how vengeful she is.

Well, for some reason, she seems to be pretty vengeful. I don't know what I did that made her so mad, but it's like she's punishing Itty to get at me.

So what's the plan? Where do you go from here?

That's the question. I took another deep breath as my eyes cut toward Myles. He was arranging a set of his alphabet letters from A to Z. Not a care in the world. *I'm working on the answer.*

NEGLECT?

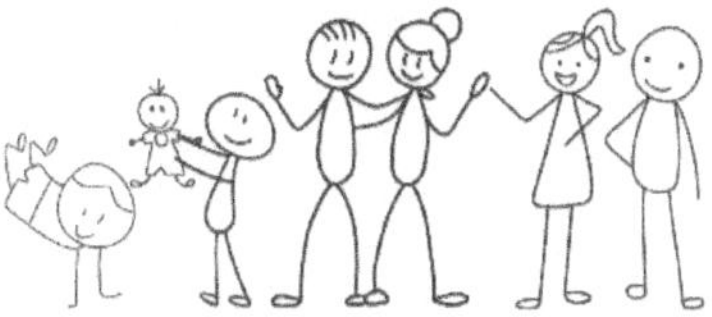

You should sue that doctor. Cash was always listening. Always taking in everything around him and analyzing it, trying to use what he knew to solve the problems of the world—and especially the problems of those he loved.

We don't want to sue *anybody* I reasoned. *A lawsuit is expensive, Plus they can take years and years to resolve, and hospitals have high-powered attorneys on staff. Regular people almost* never *win against hospitals.*

But we have to do something! He's sick almost all the time. It isn't fair for a baby *to be sick. And especially not our Itty Bear. He's just so cute and adorable. He shouldn't be sick.*

Cash was my most empathetic child. I can't count the nights he heard me or Shawn walking around with Myles and he jumped out of bed to try to help. Sometimes we could get him to go back to bed and lay down, but most nights I would say *bring him a cool washcloth* or *get us a towel*. He seemed to be able to go back to sleep after he'd done something to help.

Maxie was pretty small still—during the worst of it—and Myles' illness affected him in a different way. Well, in a few different ways. He hurt for Myles. He would say, *I'm so sad that Myles is sick. He's just so little. I don't like it when he's feeling bad. Poor Myles.* Maxie was so little, too, and he had the sweetest, softest little voice. When he would talk about his baby brother being sick, it would break your heart.

When you have multiple children, (*especially* when most of them are surprises) there is a period of time when each one is the baby. This was particularly true of Max—he was our *last* baby. We really thought he was going to be the permanent baby of the family. And then, he wasn't.

When I went to the hospital to deliver Hailey and Caleb, the standard stay was a *minimum* of two nights. It gave the mom and baby a little recovery time, and allowed baby to be monitored for any conditions that would appear after birth. When I had Cash, they kept us for two nights, but we were out as soon as they could serve the discharge papers that second morning. Only three years later, I had Max. Apparently, July 2015 was a very prolific time, because they were ready to boot us out as soon as 24 hours was up so they could fill the room with new occupants. Fast forward three more years, and it was time for one last trip to the maternity ward. This time, I don't think we made the 24-hour mark. Nevertheless, my hospital stay with Myles (the first one--when he was born) had a lasting impact on Max. To this day, he will say *I didn't like it when you left me to stay at the hospital. I really missed you.* He was safe at home with his daddy and Cash, but he had never spent a night away from me. I missed him every bit as much as he missed me, but that hospital stay changed his position from *baby* to *big brother*, so it was truly a life-changing event for Max.

Although Maxie loved the new part he played in the family, it *was* a pretty big adjustment. There were never any signs of resentment or animosity towards his new baby brother. In fact, he would frequently say, *I'm so glad God sent us baby Myles.* Also, we made an extra effort to spend time with him and let him know how special he was. But after only a few weeks, Myles' symptoms began. We now had this very sick little baby. Whenever he had an episode, we would go into survival mode. Maxie shouldered right on through with the rest of us, but *I* know how much he missed out on.

Max and I had been inseparable since he was born. When Hailey and Caleb were babies, our lives were pretty tumultuous. My doctor (keep in mind, this was over twenty years ago—*very* outdated medical advice) advised me to stop nursing Hailey immediately when I discovered I was over two months pregnant with Caleb. She was barely four months old. I could give plenty of excuses for only nursing Caleb for *three weeks*—I was young....I was tired....my husband (not Shawn--this was before him) wasn't a fan of me nursing—but I still feel guilty about how quickly I stopped. Caleb had some health issues and I blamed myself for not trying harder to breastfeed him longer. So when I started having babies again in my thirties, I was determined to exclusively breastfeed, and to continue until the babies weaned themselves. And I did. Maxie was still nursing, still falling asleep in my arms, all throughout my pregnancy with Myles. And once Itty was born, I would hold them both with their feet tangled together, Max partially cradling Myles, while they ate, then drifted off to sleep.

I once had a doctor (an older one) express his shock when he found out I was still nursing Myles at barely over a year old (he would've *really* come unglued if he knew I nursed a three-year-old).

Why don't you give him real food? I can still hear the confused distress in his voice.

I do, I explained. *He eats real food... I nurse him for the connection. It's calming. For both of us.*

I could've explained to the doctor that not only is extended breastfeeding an amazing way to create a lasting bond with your child, it's also been proven to be beneficial to the mother's mental health and lowers her risk of diseases (like cancer and high blood pressure). Even more importantly, the nutrients in the milk transform to meet the child's needs so that it continues to nourish them based on their age. It's truly miraculous. And of course, there's the protection that a baby (or, *child*—depending on the age) gets from mom's antibodies. It's just an all-around good thing. (CDC, 2023)

So, I was still nursing Max when Myles was born. And we had no foreseeable end date. When Cash was three, he started falling asleep on his daddy's shoulder. He didn't ask for *booba* (that's what Cash called it) anymore, so he kind of just weaned himself. Max only nursed at night, but he didn't seem to have any plans of stopping. We figured it would just happen when it happened. Shawn loved to say—facetiously—to the boys, *when you go to school, you're too big for baboo*. I thought he was sooo funny. (Just picture me rolling my eyes here, please.) Anyway, Max was not ready to quit. But when Myles started getting sick, he needed me. During his episodes, Itty was on me ninety-nine percent of the time. It's 99 instead of one hundred because sometimes I would hand him to Shawn so I could go pee. *Sometimes*. There were many, many times he went with me—often, *latched on*. We were *all* exhausted. I was holding (and nursing) Myles around the clock. So it was pretty much a necessity to stop breastfeeding Max. I know, I know. He was three years old...

Mom guilt can be crushing. And for me—when Myles was sick—well, it was like no matter what I did, I wasn't doing enough. I was holding Myles, nursing Myles, bathing him in lukewarm baths, walking with him, singing to him... but he was still miserable, and he was still sick. That was my fault. And while I was taking care of Myles, I was completely neglecting my other children. It didn't matter that two of them were grown and the other two were getting *all* of their dad's attention. *I* was not doing what I needed to do for them. They needed their mother, and I couldn't be in two places at once. That was also my fault.

Obviously, looking back I can be kinder to myself. I know that if I was talking to someone else in the same situation, I would say *Don't be so hard on yourself! You are doing your best!* But I'm *not* talking to someone else. I'm talking about myself. My kids. So while I can reminisce and understand that I was doing the best I could do in that moment, I still feel the weight of regret. It's not as heavy. But it's still there.

When Myles was healthy, I tried to make up lost time with my other children and other responsibilities. When we came home from the hospital stay, Myles was absolutely at one hundred percent. He felt great. All was—temporarily—right with the world.

Shawn and I still woke up through the night to make sure he was okay. And I had about a million things to catch up on that I had let slide while he was sick. But it was so much better than when he *was* sick...it's like when you're living paycheck to paycheck, being completely broke for a few days, and then your money hits your bank account. You still have bills. You're definitely not rich. But for that moment, you feel like a millionaire.

So things were pretty great, but we were always waiting for the other shoe to drop. Or, more accurately, for Myles' temperature to spike. (Did you know that that expression came from when people lived in cheap tenement housing and they would hear their neighbor take off a shoe, then *wait for the other shoe to drop*? They knew it was coming.) We knew the spike was coming. We even knew *when* it was coming. But we still didn't know what to do about it.

I had, of course, continued researching fever disorders, hoping that something would pop up that would help us to help Itty. Dr. ******* was an infectious disease specialist, and while she knew what PFAPA was and claimed to understand the symptoms (her PFAPA patients *always* had mouth sores), I wasn't sure that was the right specialty for what we needed. I kept seeing the word *rheumatology* pop up. It instantly brought to mind a story my grandma had told me, when I was a child, about an elderly woman who had rheumatoid arthritis. The lady had it so bad that her hands and limbs curled up. The visceral image of the small, twisted woman, curled up into the fetal position, with her hands closed into fists that would not unclench, burned into my brain. Once, a few years ago, I was so dehydrated that my hands started to clench, and the memory of that poor woman resurfaced like a bad dream. So while the idea of anything to do with rheumatology unnerved me, I wondered if that was the direction we should be seeking.

LIKE TRYING TO STOP A HURRICANE

Two and a half weeks had passed since Itty was released from UK. That night, we went to bed knowing it was time for him to be sick. Writing that now makes me realize, yet again, just how crazy and awful this illness is. You know that it's coming and there is no way to stop it. The helplessness is overwhelming. So many times I would pray for God to take what Myles had and let me have it. I know that's not how it works. But seeing your baby so sick he can't hold his head up, throat swollen and red, *burning* hot, not able to eat... it was the worst.

And while the stay at UK is a terrible memory that I wish I could forget (kind of like some of the dates I went on in my twenties) it did do one good thing: it made me even more sure that we knew what Myles had. Two of the residents had basically told me he had PFAPA. Myles' blood labs there also supported the diagnosis. And it gave me the one last shove I needed to break it off with Dr. *******. For good.

Since we knew it was time, I kept waking up to feel Myles. He was a little more restless than usual, but he never got hot. We woke up. Went to school. Waited for Myles' temperature to spike.

I was in front of the classroom, teaching my kindergartners, when the phone dinged.

I've got to take this, I mumbled to myself. Then to my assistant, *Can you take over?*

The text was from Shawn, but I didn't even bother to read it before pressing *call.*

How's he doing? I blurted the question as soon as he answered. If he was too hot, I would get a sub and go to him.

He's fine, Shawn answered. *Are* you *okay? You don't usually call before lunch...*

The adrenaline surge that had just rushed through me left me trembling. *I...I got that text from you. Is he hot?*

No, honey, he's good. A little tired...he slept late and he's laying around. But he's not a bit warm. I just sent you a picture.

Wow. Well, I just saw that you texted and I freaked out...it's time, you know? I kept waking up all night to check him.

Me too.

During the early morning hours, I had reached out to touch Myles and my hand brushed Shawn's. Itty was curled up next to him like a little squirrel, his daddy's large hand on his back. As my fingers grazed Shawn's, his eyes popped open, *What's wrong?* That was our normal pattern. Hoping for the best but always on edge—especially when it got close to fever time.

When I walked in the door that afternoon I went straight to Myles, but I didn't touch him.

He's still doing good, mama. Go get cleaned up and you can have him.

Usually after school, I would sneak in and change clothes, wash my hands...sometimes take a bath. After I was disinfected I'd get Itty and we'd cuddle for a while. If he saw me when I first walked in, he'd usually reach out his little arms for me and I couldn't *not* reach back. But today I had to risk it. I needed to see him. We had been through this so many times before (and it was always nerve racking) but this time was different. We knew what he had and the doctor wasn't going to help. It was time for us to figure out the next step.

Myles was tired. He was laying on the couch watching a YouTube video about letters. No temp. No glassy eyes. But he wasn't *healthy* Myles either. Myles at one hundred percent was always jumping and talking and playing. He was his own warning signal: calm, tired Myles was a harbinger of hot, sick Myles.

I told you...he's okay. I know he's not real active today, but that could just be because we didn't sleep great last night...

You know what it means when he's like this. My voice was sharp, some might even call it shrew-like. But if you just add a *d* to shrew, you get *shrewd,* so...

Maybe he won't get sick this time. Maybe it's over. He could've outgrown it. He's been doing so good since you all got back from the hospital. (Just to clarify, he had been healthy for the *two weeks and four days* since we got home—not exactly an eternity.)

This was another part of our routine. Even though the fevers were on a basic schedule, it would occasionally change by a day or two. And sometimes we would do something different (like take Myles on a trip) and it seemed like the stress of that could trigger an episode. When his fever was a little off (even by a day), Shawn would take it as a sign that he was healed. I did understand—when he was healthy it was almost impossible to believe he would ever get that sick again—but I still challenged him.

Okay. Maybe you're right. I hope he never *gets sick again. But you sound like that crazy doctor. Do you* really *think it was "just a cold" when his fever was 105°s and he had no cold symptoms?*

Of course not, honey, I just meant...

He has a fever disorder! And it isn't going to get better until someone listens! I thought you understood. My voice grew angrier and louder as I continued my one-sided argument, even though I knew Shawn just didn't want him to be sick anymore. I felt like I was in a constant battle to get people to understand that Myles had something wrong (not just an earache or a cold) and one of the few people to see that was Shawn. When his hope (because of a day or two extra between fevers) seemed like doubt, I felt alone. Sometimes I expressed that fear as anger. It wasn't right and it wasn't smart, but I have learned, through the years, that at times I am neither right nor smart.

But I *was* right about Myles.

I apologized. We made up. Shawn is my best friend. We have had our ups and downs through the years, but if we didn't both have the ability to admit when we were wrong and to forgive each other easily, there wouldn't be any *through the years.* So that "argument" was over about as quickly as it began.

Besides cooking dinner, I mostly just held Myles the rest of the evening. At bedtime, we prayed, then we went to bed with a still-cool baby.

It started around four hours later.

Neither of us had slept soundly—I don't think I've slept through the night since I became a mom—but I definitely haven't since Myles was born. Every time I moved, Shawn would either jump up or ask, *You okay?*

Around one a.m., I heard Myles making a little noise—like he was swallowing over and over. By the time I twisted my legs around to get enough traction to raise him up, the vomit drenched me and Itty, along with the edge of our bed.

Shawn!

He was up and grabbing a towel before I finished saying his name.

I started towards the bathroom and we *almost* made it before he threw up in the hallway.

Get in the bath. I'll take care of the bed. Shawn's voice was drowsy, but he was able to rattle off directions robotically. This was not our first (or second, or third-ieth) rodeo.

Fortunately (or unfortunately, depending on how you look at it), we had this down. I was already stripping off my clothes and stepping into the tub with Myles. I rinsed us off as he cried. Waking up like this was hard on me, but I wasn't the one vomiting and in pain. After we were clean, I ran us some warm water and I sat and held his hot little body against me until I felt his breathing slow. Shawn brought us clean towels so I could wrap one around Itty, then he helped me to stand and got us both dried off and back into bed.

Myles' temp was 102.5.

First, I found a sub. Then, I got an appointment with Dr. Avery. She's the one who figured this out. Maybe she could help us decide where to go from here.

Myles! What are you doing here, buddy? Dr Avery addressed Itty as she walked in. She had a lilt in her voice, but her face showed concern.

I don't...know...what...to do. My voice broke unexpectedly. I swiped tears always and took a breath to steady myself. Though the situation was amplified by extreme sleep deprivation, I was not a completely crazy person. I would not lose it in a pediatrician's office.

I... I'm sorry.

No. No. Don't apologize. Dr. Avery reached for a Kleenex box as she sat down on her roly chair. The casters made an oddly comforting *clicking* sound as she moved close and handed me some tissues.

You know how sick he gets...

Though she was not there from the beginning, Dr. Avery had seen him more than any other physician. She had witnessed him at his worst.

...I thought she would finally have to help him.

Dr. Avery was quiet as I continued. She knew the "she" I was talking about.

The night we got there...a resident saw him and said, "Do you know about fever disorders?" She had seen him for TWO MINUTES. And she knew what he had from looking at his records.

*Did Dr. ******* disagree?*

*Dr. ******* wasn't there. Not then. She didn't show up until late the next day. His fever was gone by then. And do you know what she said when she did show up?*

Dr. Avery slowly shook her head from side to side. Her eyes revealed her understanding that whatever Dr. ******* said, it was not good. Not beneficial.

She said he had a cold.

A...what? A cold? The shock on her face was actually a relief for me. Dr. Avery was a professional with years of experience working with children. Her opinion mattered. It mattered a lot to me.

He had almost a 105° fever! He did not have a runny nose. Or any other "cold" symptoms. And what about those other thirty or forty times he was sick? My voice wasn't broken anymore. It was angry. Determined.

This baby has something going on, I continued, *and it isn't a cold. But that lady isn't going to help him. It's like she's trying to punish me for something. And I have no idea what I did, but she is hurting my baby because of it.*

Dr. Avery was quiet for a second as she took everything in. She inhaled, then slowly let the air out of her lungs before speaking.

No, that wasn't a cold. And I agree with you. He has all the symptoms of a fever disorder. I don't understand...

Dr. Avery's words trailed off and I could sense that she was being cautious as she spoke with me. After all, she had referred us to Dr. *******, and in her position it would be very likely that she would need to deal with her again in the future. Also, Dr Avery has always been a consummate professional—she would not drag another physician's reputation through the mud. But I could tell she was frustrated and confused about the situation, like I was. She said enough to let me know that she didn't think I was crazy. Myles had a fever disorder and Dr. ******* would not help him. Regardless of what she said or didn't say, I will never forget that Dr. Avery didn't give up on Myles.

Let's try a different direction.

Myles stirred in my arms, so I repositioned him to try to make him more comfortable. We had only been in the room for a few minutes before Dr. Avery came in, but already we were sticky with sweat.

Once I had him snug on my shoulder, she leaned forward and put her hand on his back, *Oh, Myles, you are so warm, baby.* Then she continued,

What if we try rheumatology?

She had already gotten my attention from *try a different direction*, but now I actually felt a real spark of hope. So much of the research I had poured over was either done by rheumatologists or mentioned that the patients—patients *diagnosed* with fever disorders—saw rheumatologists. The fact that she suggested sending him to that particular specialty before I brought it up...well, it just really made me feel like we were finally on the right track. But I still had a concern. And it was a pretty big one.

You know, everything I have been reading about fever disorders mentions rheumatology. I always just associated it with arthritis, I shrugged.

Well, they actually treat anything involving inflammation in the joints, the muscles....even the bones. And fever disorders have high markers for inflammation so they fit into that category.

Yeah, that actually makes sense, I acknowledged. *Even though there isn't a "test" for the fever disorders, high CRP and SED rate are good indicators. Along with the symptoms, of course. And not to dwell on the past...well, I guess that's actually exactly what I'm doing...but Myles' CRP and SED rates were extremely high at the hospital.* I couldn't stop myself from throwing that out there, even though I knew it made no difference now.

What? Dr. Avery's voice went up an octave. *And what did Dr. ******* say about that?*

Nothing. I mean, I doubt she was going to tell me. I asked—because I knew it was indicative of PFAPA—and a resident that was with her told me they were "slightly elevated." So I checked. They were slightly elevated like I'm slightly sleep-deprived.

Dr. Avery shook her head in disbelief.

I guess they were crazy high because he had a cold, I added the dig as I rolled my eyes.

Wow. I just— Again, she stopped herself.

Well...let's have a look at Myles and then we'll make a plan.

Once again, I shifted Itty. This time, I rotated him so that his back was against me, giving her easy access to examine him. When he was this hot, he just laid limp in my arms. His eyes were vacant—slightly open but not conscious of his surroundings. The change in our child—from healthy to *this*—was almost indescribable. Our "normal" Myles is a tornado. A happy, fun little tornado, whirling life into everything he touches. *This* was heartbreaking. He was no longer the storm, but more like a victim ravaged by it.

As Dr. Avery went through the motions of examining Myles, I raised my biggest concern,

*What if Dr. ******* tries to interfere with his rheumatology appointment? I mean, can she do that? Can she tell them not to accept him? Or cause problems once he's their patient?* The questions all came rolling out at once, then I felt like I was holding my breath as I waited for her answer. The idea of going to a different specialist gave me so much hope, but I couldn't stop myself from worrying about Dr. ******* interfering. She had acted like I was just some crazy parent who wanted my baby to have a rare disorder. If she convinced his *new* doctor of that, it could delay his treatment even further.

Oh, I don't think you should take him back to UK at all...I think we should try a different hospital.

Really? Well, that sounds like a great idea to me. Honestly, the thought of going back there....well, it's just not something I was looking forward to.

To be completely honest, I had nightmares about our experience at UK for weeks (well past this visit with Dr. Avery), so the relief that washed over me in that moment was significant.

I bet. Dr. Avery was nodding empathetically, *I'm sorry it was a such a bad experience. I really thought we were going to get some answers. But since that didn't work out, let's start over somewhere else.*

She rolled away, her exam finished.

There's a pediatric rheumatologist at Norton's, that's in Louisville....I've sent a few patients to her before—never for this, of course—but so far we've had good results. If you're okay with that, I can go make a call and get an appointment set up....

Yes! That sounds good. Thank you! I was so eager to try this new doctor—this *rheumatologist*—that I basically cut Dr. Avery off as she was talking. Sometimes, I get excited about a conversation and start talking over people. When I realize what I'm doing, I try to stop and remember that God gave us two ears and one mouth for a reason. This was one of those times. I resigned myself to *listen* for the rest of the visit.

Okay. I'll go see what I can do. While I'm out I'll send the nurse in to do the flu, strep, and COVID swabs. You know: all the regulars. Can't get out of here without a few tests, she smiled. *But seriously, we do need to check for those. If for no other reason than to prove he doesn't have them.*

I'm sorry little guy, she spoke to Myles, even though he was barely conscious. *We'll get you figured out.*

I nodded my head as she closed the door behind her, then I let one single tear escape before I gritted my teeth and pressed my fists against my eyes to stop the rest from falling. I didn't even know why I was crying. Relief that we were trying something different? Anger that we had to? Months ago I had thought we were so close to a solution, and now we were starting all over again. Wherever the tears were trying to come from, they would have to wait. Myles needed me right now.

Dr. Avery had gotten Itty an appointment that was just a month away. Hopefully, he would only have one more episode before seeing the new specialist. I knew there were patients waiting months for appointments, so I was determined to be thankful for the "short" wait time. And while a two-hour drive (each way) would be hard on Myles—we would need extra clothes, for sure—I had read about people who had to *move* in order to get treatment for fever disorders. They literally had to move. Like, from one country to another country. Can you imagine relocating your whole family because you couldn't get medical treatment where you lived?

The scariest—and most shocking—thing about that is that people have to travel in order to find a doctor who understands what they have and how to treat it. We live in America and it is consistently ranked in the top ten in terms of medical advancement and accessibility. In our personal experience, only about five percent of the doctors (including nurse practitioners and specialists) knew *anything* about fever disorders. If Dr. Avery hadn't had a coworker whose son had PFAPA, we might *still* be looking for a diagnosis.

We are so fortunate that God was watching over Myles the whole way. What was an awful, harrowing experience was made bearable because He is still in control. That's what gave us the hope to keep going. That, and also when your kid is sick, you don't stop until you find an answer.

IT'S THE MOST WONDERFUL TIME OF THE YEAR

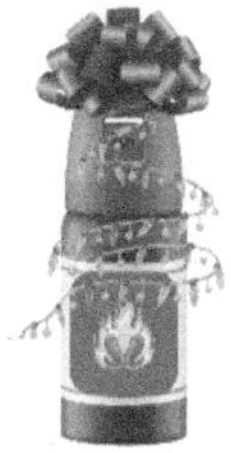

Life continued while we waited. During the good days, we decorated for Christmas, shopped for gifts online, and played catch up with all the things we pushed to the side when Itty was sick. During the bad days, we did all we could for Myles, and we survived. I remember calculating the days to see if we would be able to celebrate Christmas. It was going to be so close. Of course, we would *celebrate* either way, but would Myles be able to join in on the fun? And if the youngest member of our crew couldn't enjoy it, how would the rest of us? Only time would tell for sure.

Myles' appointment date finally came, so we loaded everyone into the van and made the trip to Louisville, home of the Kentucky Derby. This was way before our trip to California, so the abundance of the homeless population was a little shocking. There were people holding signs as soon as we exited the interstate, and others sleeping in the structure where we parked. My heart went out to them. But also, I held on tighter to Myles and had my pepper spray at the ready. I would continue to hold onto my children tightly and keep a weapon in my hand (and feel guilty about doing both) until one day in Santa Monica when Max and I were taking a walk to get snacks. The street was perpendicular to the Promenade, a very expensive, open air shopping center (think Gucci, Coach, and Tiffany) and an unhoused woman shouted, *what's your problem, b****? I'll kick your a**!* To which I quietly and quickly replied, *I don't have one,* ducked my head, and swiftly walked away—dragging Max by the hand. After that incident, I no longer feel guilty about the weapon or the child-squeezing.

In December of 2021, we were still very much under COVID guidelines, so Myles and I donned our masks while Shawn and the boys sat in the van. The offices and hospitals were connected by skywalks and the one we walked through was designed for the many children who would pass through it. It was bright and had colorful lights that moved, so as the kids passed made the walk across the bridge, they would be focused on something beautiful and happy instead of the doctors and needles ahead of them. Myles certainly enjoyed watching the mini-light show, and when he got older, he liked to chase the lights as they danced around.

The signs directed us to a bank of elevators, and there were six floors of pediatric offices to choose from. Listen, I can get lost anywhere, so this is when I *really* started to lose it. The emotional weight of the appointment was colliding with my fear of not finding our way. Fortunately, there was a super nice man at reception --we were in a big lobby, and they had what I would call a "help desk" there--and he must have seen the look of panic on my face. With a big, genuine smile he said, *Good morning, ma'am! Can I help you find what you're looking for?*

Yes, please.

Amazing what a kind act or word can do for someone. It didn't matter that he worked there. Employees overlook people all the time. This man made a conscious decision to have a positive attitude and to help someone in need. He could have just as easily ignored the fear in my eyes and looked the other way. I would've gone the wrong way, leading me down a road of negativity and lostness (Is that a word? It should be.). Instead, he helped me out, starting a chain of positivity, and we found our way. So that was nice.

This visit was not really unlike any of our other doctor visits. A friendly, young nurse took Myles' temperature, blood pressure, respiratory rate...all the vitals.

He climbed up on the scale, started reading the numbers, and didn't want to get down.

Myles, would you like to come with me?

Okay. Let's go, he said.

She took his hand and led us to the room.

Myles, she looked at him (I wonder if they teach them that? To talk to their young patients?), *have you been feeling bad?*

No, he answered.

I believe Myles thought about the sickness kind of like I did—it was hard to think about him ever being sick on the days he was healthy.

We think he has a fever disorder, I explained as she typed his information into the computer.

She asked a few more questions about his symptoms, then delivered the regular, *The doctor will be with you in a few minutes.*

I prayed as we waited. Myles squirmed. He was feeling so good. It was strange to sit in a doctor's office with this version of Myles. He seemed absolutely healthy. The week before, he was so sick that we were holding him--watching him--around the clock. Now here we were, clinging to what felt like our last hope, and you could not tell he had ever been sick. Well, except for his size. He was smaller than most one-and-a-half-year-olds. But if you didn't know his age, you couldn't tell anything had ever been wrong.

Knock. Knock.

HOW DID IT GO

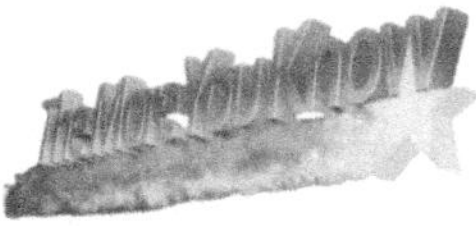

I think it went okay. I hope it went okay. I wish you could've gone with me. She was nice. Better than the last doctor. Well, an executioner would've been better than the last doctor. But, seriously, she was friendly. And she listened. She actually seemed to hear me. I guess we'll see. It's going to be okay, right?

Yes, baby. Just please calm down.

I am *calm.*

Did she tell you anything? Shawn and I had been texting all the way up until the doctor came into the room. He was anxious to find out what happened, but knew me well enough to know it would take me a few minutes to wind down and explain everything.

Well... She didn't diagnose him with PFAPA, but she didn't not *diagnose him either*, I began.

Oh great, Cash chimed in from the backseat, *another doctor who's a quack.*

Cash was the kindest, most thoughtful child you would ever meet. He was also Myles' biggest cheerleader, and the fact that Dr. ******* wouldn't help his baby brother had left a lasting impression on him.

Hold on son, I said, *let me tell you how it went first. I actually think she might help him.*

I began describing what happened starting with the nice man who steered us in the right direction, through check-in and the visit with the doctor, all the way through to searching for our vehicle in the parking structure. Spoiler alert: I gave up and called Shawn to come pick us up at the door.

Okay. Well, it sounds like she's got a lot more sense than the last doctor. I mean, we kind of knew she wouldn't walk in there and diagnose him at his first visit. I know that's what we would've liked to happen...

Yeah, I know. It's just taking so long. I guess it wouldn't have been good practice to say "Well, you're right--he has PFAPA" without doing any tests or anything. I'm just like, at this point, what else can they test? He's had more blood draws than I have in my whole life. It isn't fair.

While I did understand that going to a new doctor would mean starting all over from the beginning again, I couldn't help being disappointed that we would have to wait close to another three months to come back. And I'd be lying if I said I hadn't hoped we would leave with a diagnosis.

Baby, nothing about this is fair. But we're doing all we can. And we just have to have faith that we're finally on the right path and that this doctor is going to be the one to help him.

Shawn had not always been the one in our relationship who was all sunshine and rainbows, but he had assumed the role through this whole experience. I usually try to look at the bright side of things, but I had failed miserably at staying positive during the worst of Myles' illness. When I would get depressed about being depressed, Shawn would remind me that there had been plenty of times in the past when I had been his encourager. He said he was happy to be the strong one for me now. That was one of the great things about finding your partner in life. When I was weak, he was strong. When I started falling apart from lack of sleep, he would take the baby and send me to bed so I could recharge for a couple of hours. He always tells me that I'm the one that keeps the family going, but he's the one who keeps *me* going. I thank God for him everyday. (Go ahead and roll your eyes. But it's true.)

You're right. I know you're right, it's just...

I know. I know... It's awful. But look how strong he is. They're going to figure this out and he's gonna be stronger and tougher and, well...just look at him. He's been sick for about a third of his life and look at how good he's doing.

Shawn was right. Myles was small, but he was strong. Active. When he felt good, he gave his big brothers (and the rest of us) a run for our money. By the way...did you know that giving *a run for your money* comes from horse racing? It refers to a horse performing well for someone after receiving the financial backing from said person. And we were in horse country, so. The more you know.

It's unreal to think that just a few days ago he—

Just then my phone dinged. I glanced down at it and was surprised to see we already had an alert from MyChart.

What's wrong? Shawn was driving but he had glanced over at me when I stopped mid-sentence to look at my phone. Apparently, the look on my face was concerning.

What? Oh....nothing.... It's just....there's an alert from Myles' visit already.

I answered him absently as I quickly tried to log into the MyChart app on my phone. When I'm in a hurry, my fingers seem to stop working. It's kind of like that dream I have when I'm trying to call 911 and can't dial the right numbers.

After I *fi*nally got logged into the app (of course this was the time they wanted to use extra security: mother's maiden name...street perpendicular to the one you grew up on...first pet's blood type...click all the motorcycles that have three wheels and are driving through the stop lights), I was surprised to see several test results, as well as an after-visit report.

Well?

Just a minute, I answered him as I was quickly going back and forth between the lab results and google. I guess I had been doing that for several minutes, because Shawn asked me again,

Monica. What do the results say?

...I'm trying to figure out what Antigen Factor eight is...

What? What is that? Does he have it? Sounds like something from Star Wars...or Stranger Things...or one of those weird Broken Mirror shows...

Shawn's obvious concern and confusion made me look away from my phone for a minute to focus on answering him. I had gotten so wrapped up in figuring out what everything meant that I had forgotten how worried he was, too. I resolved to slow down and tell him what I was learning as I found it. I realized it was like when someone would say "Remind me to tell you something...I'll tell you later," which always made me crazy—I wanted to know right then.

I'm sorry. I'm just trying to cross reference the labs with what they are and what they mean. It'll probably take me a while. So far, all I can tell you is that he's anemic. We already knew he was headed in that direction...she'll probably have him start taking iron...

That's because he doesn't eat meat. And he doesn't eat anything when he's sick. I'm not surprised. He sure does eat his vegetables, though—he loves his grandma's vegetable soup—but that doesn't help his iron level. While Shawn was explaining his (probably correct) theory on Myles' low iron, I had returned to my phone to try to figure out what Factor Eight was.

Oh! Here it is... 'elevated Factor VIII is associated with an increased risk of venous thrombosis,' what the heck is 'venous thrombosis?'

Is that what he has? Shawn was panicking--just a little bit--as he drove us down the interstate.

No! I mean, that's not a disease. It's something about his blood. Maybe something to do with the anemia? I don't know. Give me a minute...

From the beginning of Myles' illness, every high and low result gave me heart palpitations. I had learned what some of the tests were over the past year and a half, but some were new and others were confusing. When I wasn't one hundred percent sure, I looked it up. I not only didn't trust the doctors anymore, I didn't trust myself.

So it says here that venous thrombosis is a blood clot that forms in a vein...

He has a blood clot? Now Shawn was in a complete state of panic. Driving our family down the interstate. Great.

No. No. Just calm down for a minute. He doesn't have a blood clot. Do I need to drive?

Yeah...because that would really make me feel better. I thought you said you didn't *want the boys to get car sick today.*

Ha ha. You're not funny.

I don't know, Shawn replied, *Some people say I'm pretty funny.*

I just rolled my eyes and continued explaining,

Venous thrombosis is *a blood clot. But, high Antigen Factor eight just means he's at a higher risk for a blood clot. Not that he* has *one.*

Okay. So we need to keep an eye on that, Shawn resolved.

Probably. At least keep it in mind.

Okay, so what else did you find out?

Well, his C-reactive protein—you remember what that is?

Yeah. I remember you telling me about that. Isn't it the one that shows he has inflammation? The one that means he has PFAPA.

Well, kind of. I mean, it does show inflammation and it's a marker for fever disorders. The symptoms and high CRP together would indicate that he has PFAPA.

Okay, so was it high?

Well, it isn't as high as when he was tested at UK...but it's over ten times higher than the top limit for normal.

What?

Yeah. But it was way higher at UK. And she said it was a cold... I couldn't help mentioning that again. That's one of those stories I'll probably be telling my great grandchildren one day... *When your grandpa was a little boy, he had a 105° fever and they told me it was a cold. Can you believe that?* Of course, by that time we'll all probably have chips that diagnose us. And I'll be so senile by then they'll just say *poor old crazy grandma... she forgot to take her medication again.*

He's just got over an episode, though. Why would he still have a high CRP?

Well...I'm not sure. Maybe the inflammation hasn't completely gone down yet? I don't know how long that takes. Even though he acts like he feels better almost as soon as it's over, apparently the inflammation lasts a little while.

Was Myles just feeling so much better than when he had a high fever that he seemed to be at 100% while he was actually still in some pain? Or did it just take time for the CRP to go down? After all, it wasn't an exact count of the inflammation, but rather a byproduct (a protein released by the liver in *response* to the high inflammation). While that could be a probable reason for the CRP to still be elevated, we would learn more about why he had that much inflammation between flares later on.

But so far the labs are still supporting the diagnosis, right?

Yes. They definitely are.

Do you think this doctor's gonna help him? Shawn asked the question that was on both of our minds.

I hope so. I really, really hope so.

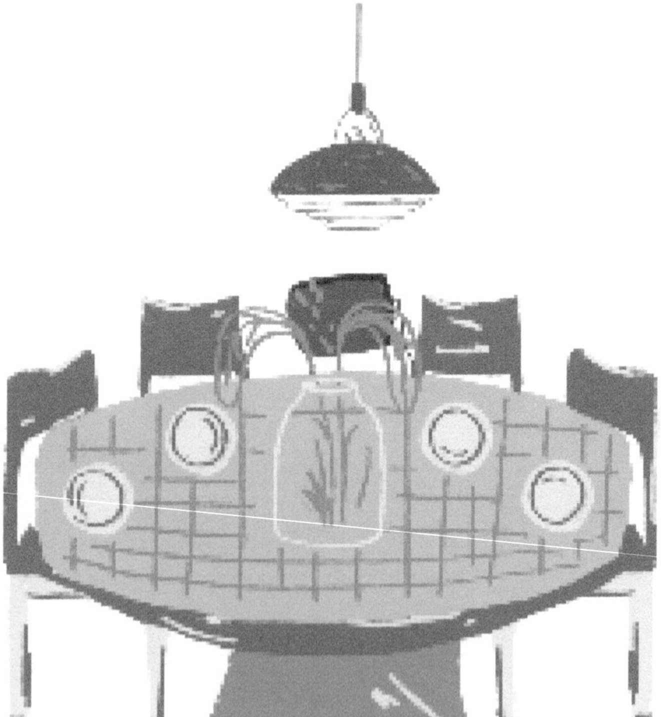

JUST A RANDOM TUESDAY

To say the following weeks were kind of busy would be like saying Johnny Cash was kind of a good singer. It was December of 2020.

Schools all over the country were trying to find the balance in keeping kids safe, maintaining their education, and satisfying parents. Our county offered classes on a modified schedule. Parents had the option of sending their children to school two days a week (either Monday/Wednesday or Tuesday/Thursday) or keeping them at home to attend virtual classes. The world was acting like teachers were on a vacation, while we were struggling to keep our heads above water. Not only did we have two groups of students to teach in-person, we had another set to teach online. We were making videos, scheduling one-on-one meets and whole group zoom-style classes, all while trying to keep our students (and our own families) safe from a deadly virus.

No one escaped the touch of COVID 19, and we each had a unique experience with it. As a teacher and a parent, the pandemic affected me differently in each capacity. We all had our own struggles; our own perspective on the pandemic and how to approach it. For Shawn and I, keeping Myles safe from the virus was paramount. We wanted to keep it far away from our whole family, of course, but he was the one who had undiagnosed health issues. Whether Myles had PFAPA or something else, COVID could be very dangerous for him.

Unfortunately, no matter how much we wanted to do everything possible to minimize the risk for Myles, not everyone in America was on board with that. (Insert shock and awe here.) The political climate turned the pandemic from a medical crisis into a divisive topic that literally split families in two.

Why are you wearing a mask?

To keep my family safe.

So you're just following the government's "rules," then? You're a sheep!

Thank you.

What do you mean, "thank you"? It wasn't a compliment.

Well, God calls his children sheep several times in the Bible, so thank you for calling me a sheep.

That's not what I meant! And you're just blindly following the people in power... I trust God *to protect me.*

So do I. But I also believe He gives us the intelligence to do things to protect ourselves. If you were drowning and someone threw you a life preserver, would you just ignore it and say, "glug... glug... I don't... glug... need...that...thing... glug...glug...glug..." Dead.

No, but... But you're twisting things around. And if it's my time to go, well then, so be it. COVID, take me home. I'll bet you're gonna be one of them vaxxers, too. Not me. I'm not going to be putting that poison in my body (as our imaginary friend takes a drag off his cigarette).

For me, it was heartbreaking to hear intelligent people, who I cared greatly about, lose their minds because of politics.

Since "COVID" showed up, nobody has a cold or the flu anymore. You could literally hear the quotation marks when they said COVID, and they seemed to be disappointed by the absence of those illnesses.

Do you think that could be because we are all separated, washing our hands more, and wearing masks?

No. It's a government conspiracy.

On the other side (the "maskers," we'll call them) I heard people say, *they're killing themselves off. They won't quarantine. They won't wear masks. Just let them thin themselves out. Seems to be what they want to do anyway.*

That is extremely wrong and very sad for two reasons. Number one, we're talking about humans. People we love. People we care about. If you see someone you love with a knife to their throat, you don't just ignore it. And secondly, their decisions put the lives of innocent people at risk. Innocent people like my one-year-old son.

Could we have kept him at home? Yes. All the time? Sure, we could have (and we did for the most part). But we couldn't keep him at home forever. And even if we could keep Myles at home, at least one of us would have to leave the house eventually to earn an income. The best way to keep Myles (and thousands of others) safe from COVID was the development of herd immunity.

I'll explain. Those who are immunocompromised—as well as very young babies—cannot get vaccinated. They rely on herd immunity to protect them from the diseases that most of us are able to get vaccinated against. Polio, smallpox, diphtheria, and rubella no longer dominate the nightmares of new parents. In fact, a lot of them only know of those diseases because they are the names of the vaccines their children get at the pediatrician's office. That is an amazing thing. And it is because of herd immunity.

Simply explained, herd immunity is when a very large sector of the population is immune to the virus or bacteria that is causing a certain disease. When the virus or bacteria has nowhere to go (because so many people are immune), it is basically eradicated. The unvaccinated are protected because of the sheer number of people who are either vaccinated or have developed an immunity due to a previous infection.

Sounds great, right? After all, look at all of those terrible diseases that have been virtually erased because of the amazing scientific breakthrough of vaccines! (By the way, if you don't want to have terrible nightmares, I would recommend that you do *not* do a google search for "diseases making a comeback due to anti-vaxxers.") So why haven't we gotten to herd immunity for COVID 19 yet?

Unfortunately, there are a few reasons. First, while there is some immunity after contracting and recovering from coronavirus, it is unknown how long it lasts. It does not give you infinite immunity against the disease. Secondly, it is possible to contract COVID after being vaccinated. The likelihood of an infection is significantly lower after being fully vaccinated (get your boosters), but it is possible. And finally, the biggest reason herd immunity has not been attained is because of politics. (This moment in time is not going to look good in the history books.)

There was so much misinformation spread about coronavirus that many people were afraid to get a vaccine. Some politicians turned the global health event into a political device to divide America. Millions of people died because of lies (6.9 million, as of November 2023). A lot of those people were good, they were intelligent, but they believed the lies that were repeated to them over and over and in many forms (television, Facebook ads, Twitter—aka *X*—, and more).

All of those things contributed to delaying the herd immunity effect for COVID 19. Fortunately, many people have now gotten the vaccine. Those who are vaccinated can get a "breakthrough" infection, but the symptoms are very mild. If you are fully vaxxed and get COVID, you don't have to worry about being put on a ventilator. Or dying. (At least, not from the COVID.)

The lifesaving COVID 19 vaccine was first available in the United States in December 2020.

Cash wanted to get vaccinated as soon as he heard it had been released. Since he was eight years old and it was only available to the elderly, those with health issues, and to medical professionals, he had to wait almost another year. Hailey, however, had started working as a phlebotomist so she was able to get a vaccine during the first round. It was obvious, before the vaccine had even been created, that it would be a while before it was widely accepted. We kept Cash and Max at home for the entire 2020-2021 school year. I wore a mask when I went to work and Shawn stayed home with the boys. Similarity to the previous year (when we thought Myles was getting sick from viruses) I would go straight to the shower when I got home in the afternoons. My clothes went directly into the washer—not in the hamper where little hands could touch them—then I could finally hug my boys. Myles and I would cuddle, then I would work with Cash and Max on their schoolwork. Eventually, I would start cooking dinner (unless I was too tired, then Shawn would make something or go through a drive through). Finally, we would clear the books and laptops and pencils from the table, and we would all sit down to dinner together.

Dinner. One of the most commonplace, mundane parts of our day. But the scene of so much love, and countless memories. And for this book, the turning point of our story.

We were sitting around the dining room table. It was one of very few pieces of furniture that was older than all of my kids. Hailey and Caleb's dad and I bought it to go in our first *real* apartment when we got married. I say *real* apartment because the *actual* first apartment was a cracker jack box; there wasn't room for a *chair*—much less a dining room table. Through the years, it has traveled with me from place to place. Once when I was in a dangerous relationship and had to get out quickly, it was one of the items I took. The setting for so many birthdays. Serious conversations. Tears and laughter. If there was a movie about my life, it would be an integral piece of the scenery. So it was fitting that we learned the truth of Myles' illness while sitting around that table.

Ding.

My phone made that familiar noise that signaled I had a new notification.

Are we ready to say prayers? Cash asked the question as I sat the remaining food on the table and made sure everyone had a fork and a drink.

Okay. I think we're ready. Go ahead, Cash. Boys, put your hands together.

Cash prayed for our meal, then we began eating and talking about our day, the *ding* (one of many that day) forgotten, until a different sound came from my phone. This time, it was alerting me to a text message. I flipped my phone over to see if it was something I needed to respond to right then, when I saw the notification for MyChart.

Hey! If mom gets her phone, then I want my phone. Max jumped on the opportunity to point out that I had looked at my phone for a second at the table, in hopes that we would give in and let him have his.

You're not getting your phone at the dinner table. Shawn is not good at saying no, but we are both resolute about that rule. Then (to me), *What's going on? Is everything okay?*

Before I could answer him, Max whined, *It's not fair!* Maxie was ready to put up a fight—usually he could get his daddy to give in to most things if he tried—but Shawn saw the look in my eyes and said, *Max. Drop it.* And Max, amazingly, dropped it.

The phone says we have test results. On MyChart. I answered my husband while logging into the app. I was curious, but not worried. This could only be the genetics panel, and it didn't test for PFAPA. I wanted to see it, even though I had looked into the diseases they were testing for and knew he didn't have any of them.

Monica? What's going on?

Shawn told me later that my face had gone completely white. This would be the perfect place for a joke about my face already being so white like, *I don't know how he could tell the difference because my face in the winter was about as white as (insert famous pale person here)* or *if I got any whiter, I'd be translucent.* I decided against it though...making a joke about skin color seems a little risky.

I know I was shaking because I remember having that feeling you get when you forget to eat. Looking back, it's kind of ironic that the two times I can remember being speechless are both because of test results linked to Myles. (The first being those two lines announcing his impending arrival.)

Shawn was waiting for me to tell him what had caused me to go mute and start trembling, so I finally just handed him the phone.

The message said:

> Patient Notified via MyChart. Genetic testing is consistent with Familial Mediterranean Fever. This disease can be inherited from parents and the lab recommends that you consider having parents tested also. He should be taking colchicine, multi-vitamin with iron and an additional iron (I am sending to pharmacy). Our clinic will call with an appointment this week as I would like to see him before the February appointment. Thank you.

While Shawn read the message the doctor had sent us alongside the test results (I hadn't even opened the *actual* results yet) I started to drift back to reality. I realized that I now had a new mission: find out what Familial Mediterranean Fever was and how that would affect the rest of Myles' life.

What does this mean? Is it bad? Shawn continued to eat as he questioned me. His eyes didn't meet mine, and I could tell he wanted to pretend that this was not a big deal.

I'm not sure.

O...kay. So... Do you know what that is? The Mediterranean Fever or whatever? Can they make it go away?

I don't exactly know. I've heard of it...I read a little about it when I was researching fever disorders. But how he has it... I just don't understand.

Yeah, I remember you mentioning some of those other disorders. They sounded terrible. I thought you said he didn't have any of those things. How does he have this?

Max was moving the food around on his plate, just waiting until he could be excused so he could get back to watching YouTube. Myles was on his second serving of green beans, using his little fingers to pick one up, nibble it until it was gone, then pick up the next one. He was oblivious to the discussion about the monumental news we had just learned about his life.

Cash, as always, was one hundred percent invested in the adult conversation.

What's going to happen to Myles? he asked in a quiet voice so as not to alarm his baby brother. *Is he going to be okay?*

Cash has always been so grown up. One day I told him, *Cash, I think you're an old soul.* When I explained what that meant, he said, *I think you may be right. Because I like old things—like wars. And people.* I often forget that he's still a child. I'm going to use that, along with the shock of seeing the consequential test results on a random Tuesday afternoon, as my excuse for being so reckless with my words in front of the boys. The tears he was trying to hold back reminded me that, old soul or not, he cared greatly about his baby brother, and I should've been more careful about how I told him. Letting him overhear Shawn and I discuss it was not the best way for him to find out that Myles had a rare genetic disorder.

Myles is going to be fine. Now we know what's causing him to be sick! I forced my voice to be upbeat and cheerful.

But is it something bad? Cash was too smart to let us placate him with fake enthusiasm.

You know, to be honest, I don't know a whole lot about it yet. But we are going to find out what it is, and what we can do about it. The good thing—the great *thing—is that now we know what's been causing Itty to be sick so often.*

Don't worry, Cash. Your mom's a genius. She won't stop until she figures out what it is and how to fix it.

I rolled my eyes and smirked, but Shawn got what he wanted—to break the tension we were all feeling. We both knew the seriousness of the situation, but being wound up and hysterical wasn't helping us, Myles, or the boys.

I may not be as smart as daddy makes me out to be, but I do know how to google. Don't worry, boys, we'll figure this out.

As I picked up my phone to type in *Familial Mediterranean Fever*, I glanced at Myles—just wiggling around, playing with the rest of his food—and something broke inside me. My throat closed up and my eyes burned. I stood up and walked the short distance to the bathroom, locked the door, and slid down the wall until I felt the hard floor beneath me. I waited for the tears to come, but they didn't. Even so, the huge weight pressing against my chest and the obstruction when I tried to swallow prevented me from attempting to stand and return to the table. It felt like my eleventh birthday party, the third one after my sister was killed. Everyone was waiting for me to go eat cake, but there was an overwhelming sadness that I couldn't explain, and I didn't want the others to see because I was supposed to be happy. Celebrating. So I hid in the bathroom.

I sat there for a while, trying to breathe deeply and slowly until I felt the tension begin to leave. Finally, I pressed my hands against the ground and pushed myself up, grabbed the doorknob, and started to walk out. And then, the tears hit. I sank back down. All of the worry, frustration, and exhaustion of the past (almost) two years combined with my newfound fear for Myles' future with this unknown illness. I just cried until I couldn't.

There's a verse in the Bible about God hearing your prayers even when you can't speak the words. When I walked out of that bathroom, I felt like the weight of the world had been lifted. The concern was still there, but it was bearable.

Now I was ready. I typed *Familial Mediterranean Fever* into my phone. It gave me an overwhelming number of results. I didn't know where to start, so I narrowed my search to *"Familial Mediterranean Fever cure."* Noooope.

Next, I searched *Familial Mediterranean Fever treatment*. That was better.

Whatever it is, it looks like it can be treated.

That's great! Right?

Yes. For sure. The stuff she mentioned in the message? That starts with a C? That's what came up when I searched treatment.

So she's already called him something in? Want me to go pick it up? We can start it tonight.

I mean, I think so. The message said something about starting... (I quickly switched over to photos, where I had taken a screenshot of the message from the doctor) *...colchicine. Wow. I just can't believe this. We finally know what's been making him sick and there's actually a way to help him.*

My dinner all but forgotten, I took in everything I could learn about FMF.

There's *a lot* to learn about FMF.

WANT TO LEARN ABOUT FMF?

I just don't know how we missed this. You researched all the fever disorders, right?

Yeah, I read about them. Most of them didn't match up to his symptoms like PFAPA did. I remember a little about the Mediterranean one, but I didn't think either one of us had any background from that area so I thought it was impossible for him to have it.

What about the symptoms? Have you found anything on that yet?

I nodded my head as I silently read from my phone.

Does it sound like him?

I mean, he has the symptoms—several of them are a lot like PFAPA—but we're not from the Mediterranean! I just don't get it! My ancestors are from Ireland! At least, I think they are...

That's where my dad's family's from, too. "O'hare." No real mystery there. And, you know my mom's grandmother was from the Blackfoot tribe. Native American is a long way from Mediterranean.

After I really dug into all the information on the disorder, I was shocked to learn that in Turkey (where the prevalence of Familial Mediterranean Fever is the highest) it occurs as frequently as one case in every 150 to 10,000 people. Astonishingly, in Armenia the carrier rate is as high as one in three (Hayrapetyan et al, 2013). While carriers are often healthy, they are able to pass on the gene mutation to their children. I was not able to find good data on how many people have FMF in the United States, but the numbers are growing. According to an article on StatPearls (Bhatt, 2023), many of those who have FMF in the U.S. are Ashkenazi Jews or people who have emigrated from the Mediterranean, the Middle East, or North Africa. Once again, none of those are true of our family. How did my son end up with this rare gene mutation?

My phone was in my hand for the rest of the night as I went through the motions of clearing the table, helping with baths, and doing whatever else needed doing. I was sitting by the tub and searching for answers. There were journal articles, but so much of that was over my head, especially back then when I was overwhelmed and just getting started.

I was typing FMF into the search bar on everything that had one: YouTube, Instagram, even Pinterest...then I typed it into Facebook. A group called *FMF and AID* popped up. This looked interesting. A group for people with FMF? I started reading the comments and was amazed by the stories of people all over the world. These were parents searching for help for their very sick children--just like me. Often, the fevers were written as celsius (because the only countries who don't use the metric system are the United States, Liberia, and Myanmar), but the fevers, the pain? It was like someone wrote Myles' story and just changed his name.

It wasn't long before I saw a post about colchicine, the medicine that was mentioned in the doctor's message. People talked about how hard it was to find (in some areas) and how expensive it was. Shawn had already gone to the Walmart pharmacy to try to pick up his prescription and they didn't have it. Now I panicked: what if now, knowing what was wrong and how to treat it, we couldn't get the medication he needed? I started searching for all I could find about colchicine. Did insurance cover it? Was it widely available in the U.S.? I found conflicting answers. I was surprised to learn that it was known as a medication for gout (the foot disease). How was foot pain related to a fever disorder? I went down another rabbit hole.

We tucked the boys in and said our prayers. This is the time I usually plug in my phone to charge it for the next day. Not tonight, though. I was lying in our king-sized bed with my phone in my hand, snuggled tightly between Max and Myles. Funny how no matter how large our mattress is, I always have just about eight inches of space. (And I wouldn't have it any other way.) Sometime in the darkness, I woke up to Shawn taking the phone out of my tightly clenched grip, *I'm going to plug this in for you*, then I fell back asleep.

When some major thing happens in your life, have you ever gone to sleep and had crazy dreams, then wake up panicked and shaking because you remember what your reality is? No? Just me?

You know, I hope you have never gone through that and never do. It's the worst.

Once, I lost someone I loved (let me just make this clear—so no one gets any crazy ideas—I am definitely *not* talking about one of my ex's), and I went to sleep and had a wonderful dream. They were with me and we had the most incredible reunion. We were happy—happier than I had been in months—and it felt so real. So. Real. Then I woke up. The joy drained out of me so fast, it was like giving Myles a glass of red kool aid and sending him into a room with white carpet. It was full on and vibrant. Then it was gone, and all that was left was devastation and heartbreak.

The night we learned about Myles' diagnoses was kind of like that. I had wild, vivid dreams...some were great (*Myles is cured!*) while others were nightmares which I will not commit to print. I would wake to reality. *We have a diagnosis!* The joy of knowing what was causing Myles to be sick for so much of his life collided with the fear of FMF and how it would affect him. The nights went on like that for a while. Even as I learned more about FMF, I would be comforted in knowing we had a plan, then crash into the depression that he could one day have devastating consequences from this disease. In the worst of times, I would not only fear the unknown, but I would mourn the lost days of the past. Why didn't I do more, sooner? Why didn't I ask for genetic testing earlier? How did I miss this?

In times of trouble, we turn to God. As I've traveled through life (yes, I could've just said *aged*, but no, thank you), I have learned to thank God for all the good He has blessed me with. Still, it is in the pain when we cling to Him. Our struggles nudge us toward His word. Require us to lean on Him. He is our comforter. I think back to watching Myles suffer, and how I would have done anything to help him. God loves us so much, that He gave his own son to suffer. To die. For all of us. I have no words that could do that justice.

God not only offers us eternal peace in Heaven, He helps us every day here on earth. Psalm 120:1 *I call on the Lord in my distress, and He answers me.* And believe me, I called on Him. And He answered.

Once, when I was at the lowest point in my life, I wanted to die. I was afraid to kill myself—I knew it was wrong. I prayed and begged God to fix what *I* wanted fixed. He had a different plan. I found out I was pregnant with Cash. It shouldn't have been possible, but with God...

My point is, he knows better than us. We may not even realize he's answering our prayers until we look back days, weeks, even years later. And he answers in different ways. When I look back on the beginning of Myles being sick, all the way through figuring out how to help him, I can see how God put certain people in my life, and he did so many things that I didn't even notice back then to take care of Myles and our family. God is so good!

I had felt helpless for so long. Now I had something substantial to do for Myles. I read the research. Looking back to those early days, I remember the times I complained, reasoned, or explained whatever new article I had been reading to Shawn. I wanted everything to make sense—to fit like a puzzle—but I was having trouble putting it all together.

As I mentioned before, a lot of the information I read was over my head. I do not have any sort of medical background, although, when I was a child, I interviewed the doctor that lived across the street from us because I wanted to become a neurosurgeon. (He had sewed up my face when I went a little too hard on my Spider-Man bouncy ball and bounced right into the wooden frame of our television set...it was the 80's.) By the time I actually started college, I had other things on my mind. So beginning with a layperson's knowledge base, I read—and tried to understand—as much as I could. I would read, Shawn and I would assimilate the information to the best of our abilities, then I would read some more. Having someone to discuss the new information with allowed me to have a better comprehension of what I was reading, but we're still talking about medical journal articles written by doctors, many of them with specialties and years of education and research under their belts. If we were having this much trouble with understanding what was written about our son's illness, how would someone with little to no education understand it?

The FMF and AID Facebook group was, without a doubt, the best place to find usable information that I could easily understand. I could ask questions and get answers. The Facebook group was where I learned I needed to cut out dairy while giving Myles colchicine. (This isn't true for everyone, but he was having stomach issues so eliminating dairy was the first step in trying to get him to tolerate the medication.)

In the group, I also learned that FMF was actually diagnosed clinically rather than based solely on laboratory testing. Myles, of course, received his diagnosis after genetic testing found a mutation in the MEFV gene, but you don't *have* to have a mutation to be diagnosed. This was talked about within the group, but I found the support for it and the details in journal articles.

It's actually quite interesting how the FMF diagnostics is formulated. (Disclosure: *I* found it interesting, but you may compare it to watching paint dry. When your kid has a rare disorder, you tend to find any information about it *interesting*.) Also, everyone doesn't use the same criteria to diagnose FMF, but this seems to be the most widely accepted one. There is a chart called the Tel-

Hashomer clinical diagnostic criteria. Essentially, the physician examines the patient and asks about their symptoms and family history, and then that is cross-referenced with the Tel-Hashomer criteria. To consider a diagnosis as positive for FMF, the patient must meet certain requirements. If he or she has two or more major symptoms *or* one major and two minor symptoms, they are considered to have FMF. The major symptoms include: recurrent febrile episodes with serositis, presence of amyloidosis, and response to colchicine. (Bashardoust, 2015).

Let's break that down a little. Recurrent means it happens repeatedly, specifically (in regard to this criteria) it must be at least three episodes. By the time Myles was diagnosed, he'd had around forty attacks. Febrile refers to having a fever. The fever must be greater than or equal to 38° Celsius (that's 100.4° Fahrenheit for us Americans). Myles unfortunately aced this part too: his fever ranged from 102.5 °F to 105.8 °F. The last word of that first category got me: serositis. Thankfully, I've got the internet. Serositis involves inflammation of the membranes which line the lungs, heart, and abdominal cavity. If I'm understanding correctly, this is where the pain comes from. Myles wouldn't really tell me where he was hurting, but he would cry out, especially while he was sleeping. He would also draw his knees up like his stomach hurt.

The second major category, presence of amyloidosis, is something that (thankfully) doesn't happen to all people who have FMF. When someone has an FMF attack, their body can produce a protein called Amyloid A. Sometimes, this protein builds up in the organs and impairs their ability to function. Kidneys are the most common target, and as you are probably aware, renal failure is no joke. While the fever episodes can make someone feel absolutely miserable, the silent buildup of Amyloid A can be fatal.

This brings us to major category number three: response to colchicine. Similarly to how a positive response to prednisone can support a diagnosis of a fever disorder, response to colchicine is a major indicator of Familial Mediterranean Fever. This simply means that if a patient begins treatment with colchicine and their inflammation, fever episodes, and/or other symptoms cease (or, at least, decrease significantly) it is a very good indication that said patient has FMF.

Now, before we dive into the minor categories of the Tel-Hashomer criteria, let's explore the link between Amyloid A and colchicine. Colchicine not only helps to prevent or reduce attacks in individuals with FMF, but it also prevents and treats amyloidosis. For this reason, many doctors recommend that all FMF patients maintain colchicine treatment, even if they are not having symptoms.

There are researchers looking for a correlation between the gene mutation and those individuals who develop amyloidosis, since it doesn't occur in all cases (Meddlej-Hashim et al., 2004). This would be beneficial for a couple of reasons. First, it would allow doctors to monitor those patients more closely and make sure they are taking colchicine daily. Secondly, it could allow certain individuals to discontinue the use of the medication.

What would be the benefit of allowing someone to discontinue the daily dose of colchicine? Well, without knowing for sure that the individual would not be likely to develop the life-threatening amyloidosis, it would *not* be worth the risk to stop the treatment. But let's imagine the research does lead doctors to know who is at risk and who isn't. Colchicine can have some pretty harsh side effects, just like many other medications. Don't get me wrong, for those who need it, colchicine is life-altering in a very good way. But there are many, many people who have stomach issues while taking it (especially at the beginning). Although most people can tolerate it after a bit, some have to cut out dairy because of the stomach pain. In addition to the side effects of the medication, there are other reasons it would be better for a person to not have to take it. Some people prefer to avoid any type of medication at all. They don't want to put anything in their body besides organic food and water. Also, colchicine is expensive (though its cost is nothing compared to the biologics—we'll get to that later). Some families struggle to purchase the medication. They may not have quality insurance, or their insurance may just not want to cover it. What do you do if you have to choose between buying your child's medicine for the month or paying rent? (And, no, I am not exaggerating. This is a real issue that some families face.) Another challenge with colchicine is the lack of availability. There was one pharmacy in our county that was able to track down the medication for Myles. Eventually, there came a time they couldn't get it. I cannot speak to the availability of colchicine everywhere, but for us (Kentucky, United States), it was a problem. If a person is not having fever episodes or experiencing any symptoms of FMF, it might make sense for them to stop taking the medication. That's if, and that's a big *if*, researchers find which individuals are most likely to experience amyloidosis.

Now we're on to the minor categories. In case I lost you there, we're still discussing the clinical diagnostic criteria for FMF. If a patient only presents with one major category, they can still be diagnosed with FMF if their symptoms align with two minor categories. The first minor category is listed in a couple of different ways, depending on the source. In the article by Bashardoust (2015), the first minor category is *recurrent febrile episodes*. The Merck Manuals website gives a slightly different designation: *incomplete attacks involving the chest, joints, or both* (Livneh et al., 1997). The data on the Merck site is taken from an older article, but the information it includes can help us understand the differentiation between the febrile episodes of the major category contrasted with those of the minor category. Basically, the *incomplete* attacks present with a normal temperature (under 38 °C, 100.4 °F) and are shorter or longer in duration than a "normal" attack.

The second minor category is *Erysipelas-like erythema*. More terminology that was way over my head. Also, I would not advise googling the above term(s) unless you're into that kind of thing. And by *that kind of thing*, I mean looking at dermatological outbreaks, because Erysipelas-like erythema is a rash which usually manifests on the lower leg/calve area. Some people refer to it as "the rash of FMF." Fortunately, Myles has skipped out on this symptom so far. I hope it stays that way.

The final minor category is the presence of *FMF in a first-degree relative.* A first-degree relative only includes the patient's parents, children, and full siblings. As FMF is an inherited disorder, having a close family member who has it is a strong indicator that the patient has it (if the individual is exhibiting symptoms).

I feel like this would be a great time to remind you that **I am not a doctor.** I am a mother, and I read a lot. If you have any symptoms of FMF, PFAFA, or *any* disorder, please see a physician. But definitely, use this knowledge, check my sources, and do your own research so you are prepared when you do see a doctor. It could change your life.

CAN WE FIX IT?

Yes, we can! (But it'll take some work.)

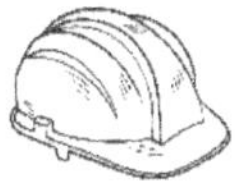

I'm going to go out on a limb here and say if we had a Mediterranean or Jewish background, Myles might have been diagnosed sooner. I say that because he fell right into many of the diagnostic criteria, but we (nor doctors) suspected the disorder because of his ancestry. Then again, there are many people (even some with the "right" origins) who have been waiting months, or even years, to be diagnosed.

The medical system is broken. Not only in America, but in places all over the world. People are not receiving the care they need.

This is partly because doctors just do not know about rare disorders, like FMF. (Do me a favor, the next time you see your doctor, ask them what they know about Familial Mediterranean Fever.) And besides FMF, there are many similar disorders that people are suffering with because the doctors don't know about them or don't understand them enough to suspect a patient has them.

I think back to Dr. ******* saying, *when you hear hoof beats, you think horses—not zebras.* Doctors are taught to think like that because they have to. If every patient who walked in with a fever or pain was subjected to testing for every rare disorder known to man, the wait time for doctors would go from hours (for a general practitioner) to days. Specialists would have years-long waitlists. But since many doctors don't even know about these disorders in the first place, the above scenario is actually an imaginary problem.

In addition to the huge issue of needing to make FMF and disorders like it much more well known, there's another roadblock to getting treatment to those who are suffering. Over and over, I encountered doctors who made me feel like they didn't believe me when I told them about Myles' symptoms, or about how often he had been sick. I get it... As a teacher, I encountered two cases of parents who *wanted* their kids to be sick. Again: I am not a doctor. These instances were both based on strong suspicions—not actual diagnosis of factitious disorder imposed on another. However, just those two occurrences had a profound effect on my worldview. I'm just saying, I can understand why a doctor (especially if they had encountered multiple cases of FDIA) would be somewhat skeptical at times. It's a sad fact that one or two bad apples can ruin the whole pie.

So how do we fix this? How do we make it possible for patients to have appropriate access to care and treatment, while not overloading the medical system anymore than it already is? It's not a quick fix. It will take a few things (and a lot of people) coming together, but if done correctly it would mean thousands of individuals would receive the correct diagnosis and gain access to treatment that could ease their suffering and, in some cases, even prolong their lives.

From our personal experience of dragging Myles from one doctor to another, combined with many, many stories of others who went through very similar circumstances, it is obvious that doctors need to be more educated about rare disorders. On average, it takes three years for a pediatric patient to be diagnosed with an autoinflammatory disorder (such as FMF or PFAPA), and it takes an average of 14 years for an adult to be diagnosed ("September," 2023).

While it is impossible for any one person to know what all of the rare disorders are, they do need to **know when to start looking away from horses and begin searching for a zebra**. If the treatment is not making the patient's symptoms go away, maybe they need to try something different. Doctors are scientists, so give them a formula to follow for when to begin looking at the more obscure illnesses.

While it seems that all of the power rests with the doctors, we have to remember that doctors are humans just like the rest of us. Some of them are incredibly amazing, self-sacrificing individuals who got into medicine because they wanted to use their God-given talents to help people. Others...well, let's just say that others had different reasons. Even those who are trying their best are still human and they may miss something. There are a few thousand rare disorders (you get different numbers depending on your source—from 1,700 to 8,000). That's a lot of disorders to remember.

When I asked Malena Vetterli, the Executive Director of the FMF and AID Global Association, what was the most important thing for people with FMF to know, she said, *They need to know how to advocate for themselves*. I wholeheartedly agree. Anyone who has (or even, believes they could have) a rare disorder needs to be able to voice their concerns to their doctor. You have to be your own advocate (or your child's advocate). The best way to do that is through education. If you or someone you love is experiencing symptoms that are not being treated (or perhaps, not being taken seriously) by a physician, do your research. Find the disorders that align with your symptoms. Once you narrow them down, read all you can about the diseases that you believe are a possibility. If you believe you could have FMF or any autoinflammatory disorder, consider contacting the FMF and AID association or visit their Facebook page to find more information and talk to people who can help you on your journey. The most important things are to educate yourself and do not be afraid to speak up.

That second one is hard for me. And I will tell you right now, if it was me with FMF (instead of Myles), it would've gone more like this:

I have a high fever and my stomach hurts.

You must have a virus, proclaims the doctor as he listens to my heartbeat. (By the way, in this make-believe scenario, this doctor is not one of the good ones.)

I had the same symptoms three weeks ago...and three weeks before...

Did you get better? The doctor interrupts me as he checks my ears.

Well, yes. But it keeps happening.

That's how viruses work. You get sick. You get better. You should think about taking vitamins and washing your hands more. His voice, exuding contempt at having to explain to an adult woman how illnesses work, let me know that the conversation was over.

And that would be it.

But it wasn't me, it was my baby. So I kept pushing.

However, if it is *you* who needs the help and you have trouble asking for that help for yourself, just remember that you deserve to be taken care of, too. God put you on this earth for a reason, and it's important to take care of yourself so you can be the best you can be. You are important.

I know. I know...that's easy for me to say (and maybe you have a healthy sense of self-worth and you are great at speaking up for yourself so it's easy for you to *do*—if so, congratulations!). But if you're like me, and questioning people (*especially* people in authority) is as appealing to you as going spelunking in the Nutty Putty cave, this next bit is for you.

First, think about *why* it's important to speak up and ask for help. Are you doing it for your child or someone else you love? Is it *you* who needs help? If it's someone you care about, just think about how much you can change their life if you are able to get them the help they need just by speaking up. If it is for you, and you *still* don't feel like your own health is important enough to ask for help, remember that by removing the barriers your illness is causing, it will enable you to be there for others, too. How many ball games or parties have you missed out on because you physically didn't feel like going? Or maybe you've stayed in bed, rather than hanging out with your family, because of pain or depression? It can be scary to speak up, but what's scarier: talking to a stranger for a few minutes, or missing out on more of your life?

Now that you have established *why* you need to advocate for yourself or your loved one, the next step is to *be prepared.* This is where the heavy lifting comes in. Research your symptoms. I mentioned this before, but you really have to dig in and find out all you can about the disorder(s) that align with what you are experiencing. I would never have been able to speak up at Myles' appointments if I had not done so much research that I was confident that he had a fever disorder. I knew what tests (and results) supported the diagnosis, and I was able to explain why I thought something was going on with him (and it wasn't a series of viruses that occurred on a schedule).

Being knowledgeable about your concerns and why they are valid helps in multiple ways. First, it will build your confidence and make it much easier for you to bring up your questions and explain your thoughts coherently. You will be able to participate in conversations with medical professionals, rather than listening passively. Having a good background knowledge also allows you to ask relevant questions while you are there with the doctor. I have learned to make a list of my questions before appointments, because no matter how prepared you are, it is usually a high-stress situation and it's easy to forget things. But, if you are already well-informed about the content you are discussing, you are more likely to think of things you want to ask *during* the visit.

Another very significant thing that occurs when you have researched your symptoms and arrive well prepared is that it builds your credibility. Doctors are more likely to take your concerns seriously if you can tell them why you believe you (or your family member) could have a rare disorder and you can back it up with facts.

Lastly, (and this is a big one) if you are an expert (or at least, well-read) in the information you are discussing with the doctor, you will know when they are feeding you B.S. At that last meeting with Dr. *******, when she told me Myles was running a 105° fever because he had a cold, I knew it was the last time we would give her any of *our* time. And while I did--somewhat--lose my temper, I was able to let her (and her people) know that I knew better by asking for his CRP and SED rates—NOT by acting like a crazy person. You get farther with intelligence than with indignation.

If the doctor you or your family member is seeing will not listen to your concerns or take them seriously, be willing to change doctors. Now, I'm not saying that if a doctor doesn't agree with you, you should just pick up and leave. Medical professionals have years of education and experience and most of them are very good at what they do. But if you feel like you are not being heard, like your concerns do not matter, you should find a new doctor. Do not pass go, do not collect $200, do not act like a Karen and get your worst moment posted on YouTube forever, just GO. Keep in mind, no matter how frustrated you are, the way you act can and will follow you. In the days of the internet, nothing you say or do will ever completely go away. There have been situations where a doctor didn't like that the patient/parents didn't agree with their opinion, so they contacted their new doctor and basically said, *Your new patient is a crazy person. Don't listen to them.* So, if you need to go, just politely leave, and find a new doctor.

When Myles was diagnosed, I was so thankful that we never gave up. We kept searching for answers and praying for God to help our baby. It was no mistake that we had taken Myles to a medical practice where someone's child had PFAPA. That led us in the right direction. Did it feel like we got derailed during the months we spent on Dr. *******? Of course it did. But I can't help but believe we went through that horrible experience so that we could share our story and help others. And, finally, we landed in the right place to get a diagnosis for Myles. This doctor was kind, professional, and compassionate. She listened to our concerns and explained Myles' condition and the implications of his diagnosis. I thank God for her and how she helped my baby.

GIRL, YOU HAVE NO FAITH IN THE MEDICINE

Myles needed colchicine to stop his fever episodes and reduce his inflammation. (And, of course, to prevent him from developing amyloidosis.) He was just under two years old when he was diagnosed, so he had been sick for one year and seven months. I should be thankful—many people go so much longer without a diagnosis—but sitting here, holding my now four-and-a-half-year-old as he sleeps, my heart hurts thinking about how sick he was those first years of his life.

We found one pharmacy who was willing to search for liquid colchicine. They found a supplier. My insurance denied the medication. It was going to be almost $500 for a one-month supply. We filed an appeal and considered paying out of pocket. It was not sustainable, but if it would make him stop suffering it would be worth it for however long we could keep it up. The pharmacist suggested we wait for the appeal, and since he was not due for a fever for two weeks, we decided to give it a few days. Fortunately, the appeal was granted quickly, and he started the daily medication.

During the first month, he had a normal fever episode. Gradually, the flares became milder. They never went away, but they were less severe—lower temps, fewer days. They were spaced out more than before. The medicine, however, made Myles have stomach issues. We took the advice of the FMF and AID members on Facebook and cut out dairy. It helped, but he still had stomach pain and diarrhea. At his worst, Myles was extremely sick for 3 to 5 days every two to three weeks, but he was thriving and energetic on the days that fell between the flares. Now, with the colchicine, he never felt *great*. He was always just a little weak...under the weather, as the saying goes. He never gained weight because he couldn't eat very much, and when he did eat, he often got sick.

Then, a whole new issue emerged. Yay.

WHAT'S SLEEP?

As problems tend to, it began in the dead of night.

I heard a noise and was reaching for Myles before my eyes were fully open. I raised him up—assuming it was the regular and we were about to be doused in vomit—but his head just rolled back, and his eyes fluttered then closed, so I laid him back down.

He must have had a nightmare, I mumbled to Shawn as I watched Itty snuggle back into a comfortable position.

Whaa... What happened? Shawn was just waking up enough to be aware that *something* was going on. I didn't really know what was happening—just that something was.

I don't know. I heard him make a noise, so I thought he was sick. Must have just been dreaming...

M'kay....you think he's alright now?

Yeah....just—You can go back to sleep. I'm being paranoid. Every little move he makes... I jump, I explained my worries away as I laid back down by Myles. My face inches from his, I was fixated on his every breath.

His breath.

Shawn. Shawn?

Yeah baby....you okay?

He's not breathing right.

What do you mean, he's not breathing right? He was now as awake as I was, laser-focused on Myles' chest.

Watch him, I said, needlessly.

We both watched as Myles breathed in and out, in and out, then stopped for a few seconds. As I started to reach for him, he suddenly took several quick breaths in—making a quick little snuffling sound. Shawn's eyes met mine for a moment, the concern in them (actually, let's be honest—it was fear) echoed my own. Then, as I looked back down, he stopped breathing again. This time, Shawn grabbed him up and said, *Myles! Myles!* And Myles cried.

From that night on, we would take turns sleeping so one of us was always watching every breath he took. (Just a side note... I'm kind of curious how many song lyrics I've written into this book by accident. Every time I do it, I get the song stuck in my head.)

We were basically zombies for the next few weeks. Even when it was my turn to sleep, I was restless. I would reach out and put my hand on Myles' belly to feel it rise and fall, then I would sleep for minutes at a time with my hand on his stomach.

Family and friends often asked how Itty was doing, so I had told a few people about his new problem: sleep apnea. Someone asked me if we had him on an oxygen monitor. It made sense. Of course, he should be on an oxygen monitor. Lack of sleep diminishes your mental acuity (as well as affecting a litany of other things). I should have already thought of getting a monitor to track Myles' breathing, but my mental acuity was diminished. Extremely diminished.

After a quick internet search, I found Owlet, a heartbeat and oxygen-level monitor that worked by using a sensor embedded in a "sock." We would wrap Myles' foot after he went to sleep, and if his pulse or O_2 dropped below a preset level, we got an alert on my phone. The first few times that alarm went off, it was a little jarring. (Imagine getting a phone call in the middle of the night: heart-racing shock.) Within a week, I was actually sleeping at night. We still took turns keeping watch, but when it was my turn to sleep, I was able to rest because I knew the alarm would alert me if anything happened.

Have you ever watched a child stop breathing? Even for a few seconds? Once, when Cash was about two months old, I woke up in the middle of the night. We co-sleep, so he was inches away from me. I watched him.

He. Was. Not. Breathing. I picked him up and yelled—actually, just like Shawn did with Myles—and he took a big breath. I think about that sometimes. God is always watching over us. Sometimes we don't realize the miracles he performs.

I don't know if the 24-hour surveillance of Myles and moving him to wake him reminded him to breathe, but it was all we could do until his new appointment. This one with a sleep specialist.

After a few weeks, we got to see the doctor and found out Myles' tonsils were enlarged. I don't know the cause (he often had a sore throat with his flares, but the sleep apnea didn't begin until he had been on colchicine for a little while and his episodes were milder), but the size of his tonsils was most likely a significant contributing factor towards his sleep apnea. The doctor wanted to perform a tonsillectomy, pending the results of a sleep study.

Myles and I packed a bag, and Shawn drove us to Louisville. We spent the night in an unfamiliar room while Myles was hooked to monitors, and videotaped as he slept.

I expected to learn the results of the sleep study the following day, or possibly a day or two later. They told me, as they hooked him up, that they would compile the data and send a report to his doctor as soon as possible.

Surprisingly, the technician came in after an hour or two. She said Myles was having over 60 apneas an hour, and she had contacted his doctor. The next morning, his doctor scheduled him for a tonsillectomy.

REMEMBER PFAPA?

So...if you're familiar with periodic fever disorders, you may already know that PFAPA is sometimes treated by performing a tonsillectomy. I don't know why it works, but (in some cases) it just does.

Knowing that it is a recognized effective treatment, you may be surprised to learn that performing a tonsillectomy (or an adenotonsillectomy—removal of the tonsils *and* adenoids) is slightly controversial when performed to treat PFAPA. Want to know why?

PFAPA, unlike other periodic disorders like FMF, almost always goes away on its own. It wreaks havoc until then...but it does eventually stop. Normally, the flares will cease sometime during the second decade of life. So the big question is: how great is the benefit of surgery versus the risk, considering that the problem is eventually going to resolve naturally?

To answer that question, you must first know the magnitude of the risks. Every surgery, whether it's a heart transplant or a BBL, comes with the potential for complications. Members of your medical care team will recite the possible dangers a few times before you go under—*just sign here, initial here, here, here, oh and the last four of your social here, and sign again—but don't worry: it's just paperwork. You're in good hands!* And, honestly, most surgeries go smoothly, just like they're supposed to. A little soreness for a few days, then you're as good as new!

There are, of course, rare occasions where complications arise. Sometimes, they are serious, but not often. Tonsil removal is different. The greatest danger of undergoing a tonsillectomy is postoperative hemorrhage (excessive bleeding). There was a study done to assess the risk for pediatric patients in which 45,940 records were analyzed from surgeries performed from the year 2000 to 2012. (Dhaduk et al., 2021) Of the surgeries performed, postoperative hemorrhage occurred in 5,470 cases. That's 11.9 percent. Wow. More than one out of ten. Now, for the sake of giving a clear, honest picture, if you do an internet search you'll get a range of data on postoperative hemorrhage. Some numbers are as low as .2 percent. I chose to share the data from Dhaduk because of the large sample size. The larger the study, the more accurate your data will be in most cases.

Three of my children have had tonsillectomies. Each time, I was very apprehensive. When Hailey had her tonsils removed, she and Caleb also had tubes placed in their ears. Hailey needed the tonsillectomy because of recurrent strep throat infections, but Caleb only needed tubes placed.

When you take a child to have a surgical procedure, a nurse will put you in a room with them where you will sign all the waivers and then wait. Eventually, they will bring your child a dose of Versed (or something similar) to make them very relaxed and sleepy, then they will take your baby from you with the promise to let you know how it's going. Tube surgery is very quick, and you get to go back to your child as soon as they start waking up.

Hailey and Caleb were both taken back for their surgeries at the same time. Caleb was done in about 15 minutes, so they let me go to him. He was a little groggy but doing fairly well for just undergoing a minor surgical procedure.

While I was sitting in the recovery room holding Caleb, I looked up as the double doors opened and saw them rolling Hailey's little hospital bed in—straight out of the operating room. That's not supposed to happen. I mean, yes, they obviously bring patients to the recovery room. But the parents aren't supposed to go back there until the child has been in recovery for a few minutes and has begun waking up. I learned why as soon as I saw her.

My heart was in pieces.

I'll try to describe how she looked, but I won't be able to do it justice. She was so little and weak from the meds. Not quite awake, but struggling to figure out where she was while she tried to pull the tubes out of her tiny body. She was bloody from the surgery (I guess they usually try to clean them up before they bring the parents back) and when I think back to that time, almost two decades ago, it still feels as though my soul is being crushed. As a mother, seeing your child like that is something you can't forget.

Hailey recovered well and had a much healthier childhood because of the surgery. But the memory of being with her in recovery has been indelibly etched in my mind.

Later, Max would need the same procedure. His tonsils were huge. The doctor took one look at his throat and said, *Ooooooh. We've gotta get those out of there.* By this time, two different people had told me about their child (grandchild, in one case) hemorrhaging days after having their tonsils removed. Getting *those things out of there* was about the very last thing I wanted to do.

Do you think, if we wait a while, his tonsils will shrink back down?

Well, when tonsils are infected—like when you have strep throat—they swell up. Then, you take antibiotics, you get better, and they go back to normal size. Make sense?

Yes.

Max's tonsils are not infected right now. If they were, I could give him some medicine, have you come back in a week or so, and it's very likely they would go back to normal.

I shook my head to let him know I was following what he was saying. *(Yes, Doctor, I understand. I'm not a complete moron.)*

Look. Right here. He waved me over and shined his bright light into Max's mouth, indicating that I should look inside. *These tonsils are abnormally large. We need to get them out of there.*

We walked out with a date for surgery for the following week.

Maxie did great. We made him drink constantly and watched him like a hawk for two weeks (hemorrhaging can occur anytime but is most common about 7 days after surgery).

Then it was Myles' turn.

Having Myles' tonsils removed, even with knowing it could possibly have the added benefit of reducing his fever episodes, was not a decision we wanted to make. But we didn't really have a choice. The child was ceasing to breathe several times an hour, all through the night. It was a case of the benefit greatly outweighing the risk.

He would be admitted to the hospital, at least one night, and they explained the extra precautions they were taking. We prayed for God to watch over him, and He did.

With each of my children, I had to weigh the benefits of the surgery and consider the possible consequences. Before Hailey, I probably knew there was a slim chance of bleeding, but I had not had personal experience with it. No one (that I knew) had told me stories about grabbing their child up and speeding toward the nearest hospital as they were gushing blood from their throat. It was not a reality in my realm of thinking, so when her doctor said a tonsillectomy would decrease her instances of strep throat, I said yes without too much hesitation. I was anxious, as any mother would be, but I wasn't *terrified*.

When you are making a decision like that, one that could end in disaster, you have to consider all sides. If I could have seen into the future—seen my tiny daughter laying there after surgery, heard the personal stories of people I knew making a mad dash to save their child's life, and learned the statistics of postoperative hemorrhaging—

would I have let Hailey have a tonsillectomy to avoid future cases of strep throat? I honestly don't know. I would have definitely been more hesitant. In Max and Myles' cases, I knew that we had to do it.

And this is why performing a tonsillectomy to prevent PFAPA is controversial. There is almost a 100 percent chance that the flares will eventually go away. You have to weigh that against the chance that during or after surgery the child could have life-threatening complications. If their case of PFAPA is very mild (few flares, short in duration and mild in intensity), it would not make sense to risk it. However, if a child was having flares like Myles did (every two to four weeks, 103° to 105° fevers regularly, not growing because the illness was so intense) I can see the possibility of leaning towards performing the surgery, just for the prevention of fever episodes. So I do understand the controversy. It's a tough decision.

Especially if you don't have all the facts.

See, I was *convinced* that Myles had PFAPA. Until I learned through the genetic testing that he had FMF, and then he got treated so I didn't think it mattered.

Surprise! You can have both.

In 2019, a study reported on the comorbidity of PFAPA and FMF. (Comorbidity just means that two diseases exist together. *Morbid* makes me think *death*, so I wanted to explain.) The study used patient data (all were diagnosed with PFAPA) from two Israeli hospitals. They found that approximately 20 percent of patients also had FMF. They concluded, *Clinicians should be aware that presentation of one disease may clinically evolve into another.* (Ariel et al., 2019)

No doctor ever actually diagnosed Myles with PFAPA, but I believe with my whole heart that he has it, along with the FMF. He had all the symptoms, and within the last year, has even had the all-important mouth sores a couple of times. I read about both disorders, and see pieces of each in Myles' symptoms. Remember when we wondered why his inflammation was high *between* flares? That happens with FMF. The abdominal pain? That's more of an FMF symptom as well. On the other side of the table, Myles often had a very sore throat with his flares, and he eventually (just a few months ago) had mouth sores.

Both disorders come with painful, awful flares, and can be treated with some of the same medications. For example, someone taking colchicine may need steroids occasionally for breakthrough flares.

But here's one reason I'm bringing all this up now. A very recent study has found that children who have a tonsillectomy for the purpose of treating PFAPA often do not have complete resolution of their symptoms *if they also have FMF*. (Gozen et al., 2023) That means, if your child has PFAPA it would be really important to know if they also have FMF before going under the knife.

NOTHING'S WORKING

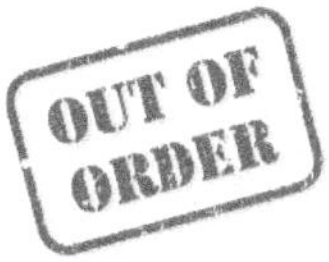

Our doctor had mentioned a drug called Anakinra early on after Myles' diagnosis. Anakinra (sold under the brand name: Kineret) is a biologic—a drug made from living organisms, such as cells or microorganisms. I was interested in this drug because Myles was struggling with the effects of the colchicine and although it dulled the flares, it didn't extinguish them by any means. Also, I had read about the difference biologics had made for some individuals and I hoped it could be the answer we needed.

As it turns out, although colchicine is the gold standard treatment for FMF, there is a small sector of patients who are considered *colchicine-resistant.* According to a study done on colchicine-resistance, approximately one-third of those with FMF only experience partial remission of symptoms while taking the medication. (Myles fit in that category.) In addition, 5 to 10 percent of patients are considered non-responders, meaning the medication just does nothing to help reduce their inflammation or halt their other symptoms. There is an even smaller percentage of the FMF population (2 to 5 percent) who are unable to continue treatment with colchicine due to intolerance of the drug, primarily because of the gastrointestinal symptoms it causes for those individuals. (Myles also fit into this category.) (Hasbani et al., 2019)

Because the medication was not working as well as it should for Itty, and he was having some pretty unpleasant side effects, his doctor made the decision to prescribe Anakinra.

So...we started the new medication and Myles was cured!

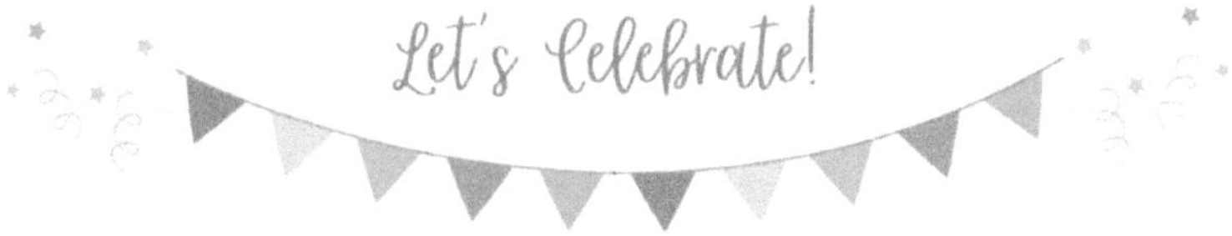

Did I get you that time? Did you really think something went that smoothly with no kinks or sidetracks or problems? Not in this story.

So, what really happened was...the insurance denied the medication. Their reason? Anakinra (Kineret) is not an approved medication for Familial Mediterranean Fever in the U.S. Even though it's been proven to help people with FMF, it does not have approval to be used for that purpose here in America, so the insurance won't pay for it.

When colchicine was denied, we considered paying the huge price so Myles could feel better. Anakinra doesn't have a huge price. It has an *astronomical* price. So paying out of pocket was not an option. (I've seen it listed at anywhere from $1,500 to $3,000 per month). There were also some drawbacks to starting Myles on this medication, as well. Number one: it was a *daily* shot. He was a toddler at the time. How many parents out there would enjoy giving your toddler a shot every single day? I was not looking forward to it.

Number two: these drugs, while usually very effective at alleviating FMF symptoms, suppress the immune response (Kineret, 2023). This makes it easier for the recipient to catch illnesses, and it means that minor infections can sometimes become life-threatening. *We were in the middle of a pandemic.* And it is for those two reasons that we didn't fight harder to make the insurance pay for Myles' Anakinra prescription. We just stayed on the colchicine train a few months longer. Until the train ran out of gas. Or whatever it is trains run on these days.

It was December 4, 2021. Exactly one year from the date of the first visit with the doctor who diagnosed Myles with FMF and started him on colchicine. The pharmacist called me. She had done her best to supply Myles' medication each month, but it had gotten harder and harder to locate, and now none of the suppliers had it. It's the kind of problem you don't really expect to have in America.

This was another one of those times when I should have had faith instead of fear.

What are we going to do?

Well, we're going to let his doctor know. See what she says about it. Shawn was calm and it annoyed me.

How can it be this hard to find something that will help Itty get better?

Why don't you look online? I'll bet you can find colchicine and order it.

What's the point? It only helps a little, and now he feels bad all *the time.*

Just give up, I guess.

I growled at Shawn as I stomped off. He knew he could make me angry enough to fix our problem.

AND WE HAVE A WINNER

(For real this time)

By the time Colchicine became unavailable, Myles had already had his tonsillectomy. We had hoped it might help stop the flares, but it didn't. (I didn't know about the study showing that a tonsillectomy often wasn't very effective in kids with both PFAPA and FMF when he had his done.) It was, however, transformative for his sleep apnea. He could breathe so much better (which is very important) and we could sleep. At least, we could sleep better than before. (Not nearly as important as his breathing, but a nice luxury and welcomed byproduct of the surgery.)

I contacted Myles' APRN. I told her we had to try something else. I knew there were other options (the doctor who had actually diagnosed Myles had left the practice, but she had told me about Anakinra and other medications that we could try if Colchicine didn't work.)

The new doctor decided to try to get Anakinra again.

While I dreaded the daily shots and lowered immunity, Myles couldn't keep going on like this. He was sick so often and he still wasn't growing.

As it turned out, it didn't matter how I felt about it. We were denied, again.

To this day, I am thankful to God that we were denied.

Because then, the doctor prescribed Ilaris. And it changed our lives.

Ilaris (or Canakinumab) is a biologic injection. It works, similarly to Anakinra, by blocking the interleukin-1 receptors that are involved in the process of inflammation. It was first FDA approved on June 18, 2009. It was not approved for use in FMF patients until 2016. Unlike Anakinra, it has a longer half-life and only needs to be administered once every four weeks (in most cases).

Myles received his first injection of Ilaris about a month before we had planned to fly to Washington, D.C. for a family vacation. It had been a few months since we weren't able to get Colchicine, so he had not had any medication during that time. The system is broken. Just in case I haven't already made that point clear.

While we hoped this was the cure we had been looking for, we had hit so many roadblocks in the past that it was hard to be too optimistic. In addition to his "scheduled" fever episodes, certain things (like traveling) often triggered a flare. This would be a risk, but we wanted the kids to experience new places and things, so we were taking a chance.

Miraculously, we made the trip, explored the nation's capitol city, and got home with no issues. As soon as we got back, it was time for his second shot.

Over the first two or three months, Myles had a couple of episodes, but they were mild. Soon, the flares were basically a thing of the past. Myles had days where he felt bad and had stomach aches, but that was nothing compared to the 3 to 6 (occasionally, 7) days of high fevers and a lifeless baby.

Ilaris has made such a difference in Myles' life. He's able to play and grow and just enjoy being a child. I ask him sometimes if he remembers when he was so sick and, thankfully, he says, *I'm not sick! I am full of energy because feel my muscles!*

He has grown some, over the past months. We believe that's why he's been having some breakthrough flares (though not like before) and experiencing occasional symptoms—the dosage is based on weight. If your weight increases, you need more medication. His doctor recently increased his dosage, so that should level him out soon. I am tremendously thankful that the worst part of his illness is now a bad memory. I hope it stays that way.

THE HIGH COST OF LIVING

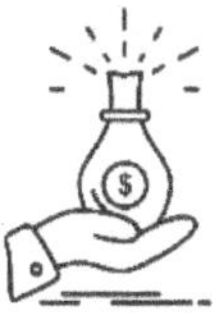

Myles is able to live like a normal, healthy little boy because he gets an injection of Ilaris every four weeks. Because over the years, there were people who cared enough to research and experiment and make a drug that would help him. Because someone (*actually*, many, many someones) cared enough to fund the research. He's able to play and laugh every day (not just some days) because there were doctors who learned about rare disorders, and one of them diagnosed him. Because the FDA approved the medication, and the insurance did, too. (Ilaris is listed as $18,765 *per shot* according to drugs.com, so we couldn't even *think* about paying for it ourselves. That is the cost every four weeks.) So many things had to come together for my little boy to be able to live a normal life. I thank God that they did.

When I reflect on how blessed we are, sometimes I can't help but think about the what ifs. What if the medicine hadn't worked for Myles? What if he had been born any other time in history? Biologics like Ilaris wouldn't be an option. And the worst, most dreadful one: what if one of those high fever episodes had taken my baby away?

I grew up in a small town—lived in the same house until I went to college, but Shawn lived all over the place. The funny thing is, he had family that lived in that same small town I grew up in. They were there years before I was even a glimmer in my daddy's eye. Well, one day when we were in that small town, we decided to drive around and see where Shawn's long-gone family had lived. We came upon the Hare cemetery.

There were *So. Many. Babies.*

Now, I am aware that the life expectancy of children was not great back then. (We're talking about the late 1800's to mid-1900's.) I can't help but wonder if some of those little ones (from infants only months old up to children a few years old) could've had what Myles had. It's genetic. We're pretty sure Shawn has a fever disorder (from looking back at his childhood—knowing what we know now), so it makes sense that his ancestors would have had cases. Back then, they didn't have treatments. They couldn't remove tonsils. (Well, they occasionally *did*—but just google the tool they used to do it with. It's barbaric.) There was no oxygen monitor to alert parents if a child stopped breathing. Obviously, they didn't have colchicine, prednisone, or biologics of any kind.

We are extremely blessed to have those medications available to us now, that people in all the centuries before us could not have dreamed about. I think about the suffering thousands of children experienced through the years... It is heart-wrenching.

But now, we have treatments. You and I can work together to make sure other children and adults don't spend huge portions of their lives in pain. We only get a little while on this earth. We should use each moment of the time we do get to make a positive impact anywhere we can. You can't do that if you're in extreme pain for days at a time. You can't do that if your child is laying lifelessly in your arms, and you feel completely, utterly, helpless. Those of us who have been blessed with good health should use some of our precious time to help other people be able to live their lives, too.

The suffering Myles experienced from the time he was three months old until he was three years old is something I pray no other child has to experience. Right now, there *are* babies, toddlers, children, teenagers, young adults, middle-aged adults, and elderly people who are dealing with one of over forty autoinflammatory disorders (FMF, PFAPA, TRAPS, HIDS, CAPS, and others).

Researchers are learning more about these disorders and the gene mutations associated with them all the time. This research will make it easier to identify when a patient has one of these disorders, and which disorder they have. Even now, we are not 100 percent sure that Myles has the exact diagnosis of FMF. There are tiny differences in some of the disorders, and the number of doctors who are actual experts and can differentiate between them is small. Right now we are just extremely thankful that he has the medication he needs, and we pray that it continues to work for him through the years.

His future is always on my mind.

Until things improve, I will be concerned about Myles' future. (Who am I kidding? I'm his mom, I'll always be concerned about Myles' future.) Not *worried*—I know God will take care of him. But until things are how they should be, I cannot stop working to fix them.

WHAT WE CAN DO

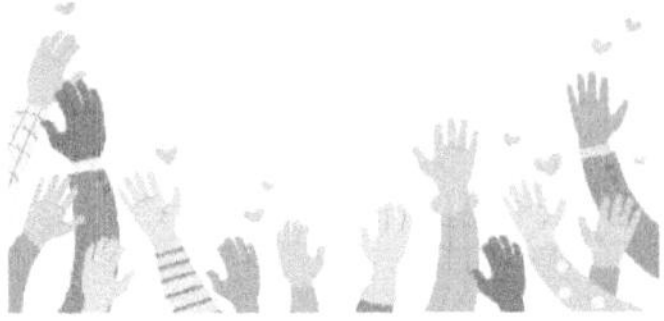

The number of people with FMF and other autoinflammatory disorders (AID) is escalating. I was surprised to learn that the state I live in—Kentucky—has a rapidly increasing AID population because of the backgrounds of those who live here. Several other states are right there with us. All over the world, FMF and AID are affecting groups that never thought they could have those disorders. Just like Shawn and I thought Myles wasn't at risk because we don't have ancestors from the Mediterranean, many doctors currently hold that same belief. In our global world, we make babies with people from everywhere. They grow up and make babies with other people. The current genetic pool is so diverse, and it will only grow in complexity.

It is very likely that someone you know (and maybe even someone you care about) has an autoinflammatory disorder. Look for the signs: fever (either on a regular schedule or seemingly caused by things like change in temperature, overexertion, or stress), joint pain, stomach pain, rashes, or mouth sores. If you have questions, ask until you get answers. Request genetic testing. But also, don't rely *solely* on genetic testing.

These are not simple disorders. Even if you find a true expert, it may take a while to determine what disorder you have and what treatment will help.

If you are able, support the research. Past research is a big part of the reason Myles and thousands of others are able to live normal lives. Although...if you've met Myles, I'm not sure you would use "normal" and "Myles" in the same sentence. Despite the danger the fevers put him in over and over, Myles is smart, playful, funny, and makes his own party wherever he goes. He was reading before he was two years old. He chases his older, bigger brothers around the house. He is mischievous, but loving. If I'm bragging, I'm bragging on our incredible Father in Heaven. He watched over him and not only kept him alive, he made him thrive.

Pray for the patients, doctors, nurses, researchers, families, geneticists, and others who are working to help others and to learn more about rare disorders.

Please, please help us spread information about Familial Mediterranean Fever and all of the autoinflammatory disorders. When even the doctors don't know what a disorder is, that is a problem. We can fix that,

together. Share Myles' story. Tell people about periodic fever disorders. Share YOUR story.

Spreading awareness is how we prevent others from going through months or years of what Myles went through.

Thank you for going on this journey with me. Together, we can make a difference for thousands of people. Remember, don't always expect horses.

Search for the zebras.

If you or a loved one are experiencing symptoms of FMF or Autoinflammatory disorders, FMF & AID is here to help.

FMF & AID Global Association is a non-profit organization that is currently helping over 100,000 patients in 54 countries, and in multiple languages.

They provide support, guidance, and information to patients and the medical community by:

- Helping patients to access life-changing medications
- Providing medical and travel assistance to patients who cannot access specialized care
- Organizing educational webinars on autoinflammation for physicians
- Connecting patients with doctors who are educated about autoinflammatory disorders
- Offering online play therapy for children with these disorders
- Spreading awareness to other families, to ensure that no child has to endure what Myles and many others like him have experienced

To learn more about AUTOINFLAMMATORY DISEASES, or if you are interested in making a donation, please visit their website:

fmfandaid.org

or

fmfandaid.org/donate

NOTES

How do I know things still need fixing? The story of Myles is just about one child. Some of this I have mentioned before but it's how I know the whole system needs to be repaired.

- Every day, more people suffer with autoinflammatory disorders.
- Doctors and hospitals don't know what these disorders are or how to treat them. If you or your child go to the ER for severe pain (women have described some of the flares as *more painful than childbirth contractions*), they are likely to label you as drug-seeking and send you home untreated.
- The average time it takes for a child to be diagnosed is THREE YEARS.
- The average time it takes an adult to be diagnosed is FOURTEEN YEARS.
- The medications are often hard to acquire in three ways: being diagnosed and receiving a prescription, having the insurance or financial ability to afford them, and the basic lack of availability.
- Some of the doctors who are actually aware of these disorders remain undereducated about them. They

want to only rely on genetics, or will not order genetic testing, or won't diagnose because of a missing symptom or unexpected cultural background.

- Ilaris (cost: over $18,000) comes in a vial containing about three times what Myles currently receives. The excess is thrown away.
- There are children and adults who have been diagnosed but cannot access the medication that would change their lives. As mentioned above: *We throw away around two-thirds of an $18,000 vial every four weeks.* How many other people do this? And, *why*?
- Many people with FMF have been misdiagnosed with appendicitis (often resulting in unneeded surgery) or rheumatic fever before receiving their FMF diagnosis.
- Specialists who have studied the research know that FMF and other Autoinflammatory disorders should be diagnosed clinically—not solely on genetics. Though there have been advances in genetic mutation research, they expect to learn about new mutations in the future. Also, research shows that 10

to 20 percent of patients with FMF have no MEFV mutation at all (Ben-Zvi, 2015).

- Recently, we had to see a doctor who was filling in for Myles' ARPN. He walked in and said, *You know, his mutation is benign.* We did not go back to him, but if we can still come across doctors who think like that--even after Myles was diagnosed based on a mutation of the MEFV gene *and* based on symptoms *and* confirmed by the significant resolution of symptoms with the use of Ilaris--**I cannot stop**.

References

Bashardoust, B. (2015). Familial Mediterranean fever; diagnosis, treatment, and complications. *Journal of Nephropharmacology*, *4*(1), 5–8. https://www.ncbi.nlm.nih.gov/pmc/articles/PMC5297479

Ben-Zvi, I., Herskovizh, C., Kukuy, O., Kassel, Y., Grossman, C., & Livneh, A. (2015). Familial mediterranean fever without MEFV mutations: A case–control study. *Orphanet Journal of Rare Diseases*, *10*(1). https://doi.org/10.1186/s13023-015-0252-7

Bhatt, H., & Cascella, M. (2023). Familial Mediterranean Fever. In *StatPearls*. StatPearls Publishing.

Butbul Aviel, Y., Harel, L., Abu Rumi, M., Brik, R., Hezkelo, N., Ohana, O., & Amarilyo, G. (2019). Familial mediterranean fever is commonly diagnosed in children in Israel with periodic fever aphthous stomatitis, pharyngitis, and Adenitis syndrome. *The Journal of Pediatrics*, *204*, 270–274. https://doi.org/10.1016/j.jpeds.2018.08.080

Centers for Disease Control and Prevention. (2023, September 7). *Breastfeeding benefits both baby and mom*. Centers for

Disease Control and Prevention. https://www.cdc.gov/nccdphp/dnpao/features/breastfeeding-benefits/index.html

Dhaduk, N., Rodgers, A., Govindan, A., & Kalyoussef, E. (2021). Post-Tonsillectomy Bleeding: A National Perspective. *The Annals of otology, rhinology, and laryngology*, *130*(8), 941–947. https://doi.org/10.1177/0003489420987438

Ferreira Cristina, S., Costa, A., Toscano, M., Kakoo Brioso, E., & Cipriano, P. (2021). Periodic fever, aphthous stomatitis, pharyngitis, and cervical adenitis syndrome: A rare etiology of fever in adults. *Cureus*. https://doi.org/10.7759/cureus.14749

Gozen, E. D., Yildiz, M., Kara, S., Tevetoglu, F., Haslak, F., Adrovic, A., Sahin, S., Barut, K., Ulkersoy, İ., Gücüyener, N., Gunalp, A., Yener, H. M., Ada, M., & Kasapcopur, O. (2023). Long-term efficacy of tonsillectomy/adenotonsillectomy in patients with periodic fever aphthous stomatitis pharyngitis adenitis syndrome with special emphasis on co-existence of familial Mediterranean fever. *Rheumatology international*, *43*(1), 137–145. https://doi.org/10.1007/s00296-022-05210-4

Hayrapetyan, H., Amaryan, G., Yeghiazaryan, A., & Sarkisian, T. (2013). PW01-034 – clinical-genetic investigation of FMF in Armenia. *Pediatric Rheumatology*, *11*(S1). https://doi.org/10.1186/1546-0096-11-s1-a87

Ilaris prices, coupons, Copay & Patient Assistance. Drugs.com. (n.d.). https://www.drugs.com/price-guide/ilaris#:~:text=The%20cost%20for%20Ilaris%20subcutaneous,on%20the%20pharmacy%20you%20visit

Kineret (Anakinra): Uses, side effects, dosage & reviews. GoodRx. (2023, February 16). https://www.goodrx.com/kineret/what-is

Livneh, A., Langevitz, P., Zemer, D., Zaks, N., Kees, S., Lidar, T., Migdal, A., Padeh, S., & Pras, M. (1997). Criteria for the diagnosis of familial Mediterranean fever. *Arthritis and rheumatism*, *40*(10), 1879–1885. https://doi.org/10.1002/art.1780401023

Medlej-Hashim, M., Delague, V., Chouery, E., Salem, N., Rawashdeh, M., Lefranc, G., Loiselet, J., & Mégarbané, A. (2004). Amyloidosis in familial Mediterranean fever patients: Correlation with MEFV genotype and SAA1 and mica polymorphisms effects. *BMC Medical Genetics*, *5*(1). https://doi.org/10.1186/1471-2350-5-4

Merriam-Webster. (n.d.). Habituation. In Merriam-Webster.com dictionary. Retrieved January 15, 2024, from https://www.merriam-webster.com/dictionary/habituation

*Table: Tel Hashomer criteria for the diagnosis of familial Mediterranean fever**. Merck Manuals Professional Edition. (n.d.). https://www.merckmanuals.com/professional/multimedia/table/tel-hashomer-criteria-for-the-diagnosis-of-familial-mediterranean-fever#:~:text=Minor%20Criteria&text=‡%20Incomplete%20attacks%20are%20painful,no%20more%20than%201%20week.

Vanoni, F., Theodoropoulou, K., & Hofer, M. (2016). PFAPA Syndrome: A review on treatment and outcome. *Pediatric Rheumatology*, *14*(1). https://doi.org/10.1186/s12969-016-0101-9

Vetterli, M. (Ed.). (2023). September World autoinflammatory awareness month. *Autoinflammatory Magazine*, *1*(3), 14.

Wang, A., Manthiram, K., Dedeoglu, F., & Licameli, G. R. (2021). Periodic fever, aphthous stomatitis, pharyngitis, and Adenitis (PFAPA) syndrome: A Review. *World Journal of Otorhinolaryngology - Head and Neck Surgery*, *7*(3), 166–173. https://doi.org/10.1016/j.wjorl.2021.05.004

Thank you for reading

SEARCHING for a ZEBRA

If you can take a couple of minutes to leave a review, I would appreciate it so much. **Your review** can help Myles' story reach others who may need it. Thank you!

Love,

Monica Hare

SearchingForAZebra@outlook.com

Made in United States
Cleveland, OH
05 November 2026

47645288R00178